P9-CDH-407

THE NEW RULES OF POSTURE

"Mary Bond's talent and expertise extended my professional dance career until age 52! Anyone who suffers from body dysfunction and pain must read her book. Actually, it should be mandatory reading for all institutions offering anatomy, kinesiology, and medical courses."

BONNIE ODA HOMSEY,
FORMER MEMBER OF THE MARTHA GRAHAM DANCE COMPANY AND
ARTISTIC DIRECTOR OF AMERICAN REPERTORY DANCE COMPANY

"I have long searched for a book that addresses the human body as a whole, and with clarity, guidance, and completeness. This book is a multi-faceted gem offering all of that and much more. I highly recommend it to teachers of movement and to anyone eager to learn how to become a better occupant of their body."

MARIE-JOSÉ BLOM-LAWRENCE,
PILATES SPECIALIST AND PROFESSOR OF ANATOMY AND PHYSIOLOGY,
DEPARTMENT OF DANCE, SOUTHERN CALIFORNIA
LOYOLA MARYMOUNT UNIVERSITY

"At last, at any level of knowledge of the body and movement, everyone will have the joy of a discovery that can profoundly change our relationship to ourselves, to others, and to the beauty of the world."

HUBERT GODARD, PH.D.,
PROFESSOR OF MOVEMENT AND RESEARCH,
UNIVERSITY OF PARIS

MAY 2007

THE NEW RULES OF POSTURE

HOW TO SIT, STAND, AND MOVE IN THE MODERN WORLD

MARY BOND

Illustrated by Stephen P. Miller

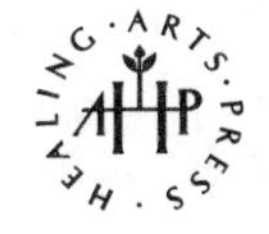

Healing Arts Press
Rochester, Vermont

NORTHPORT PUBLIC LIBRARY
NORTHPORT, NEW YORK

Healing Arts Press
One Park Street
Rochester, Vermont 05767
www.HealingArtsPress.com

Healing Arts Press is a division of Inner Traditions International

Copyright © 2007 by Mary Bond

All rights reserved. No part of this book may be reproduced or utilized in any form or by any means, electronic or mechanical, including photocopying, recording, or by any information storage and retrieval system, without permission in writing from the publisher.

Note to the reader: *This book is intended as an informational guide. The remedies, approaches, and techniques described herein are meant to supplement, and not to be a substitute for, professional medical care or treatment. They should not be used to treat a serious ailment without prior consultation with a qualified health care professional.*

Library of Congress Cataloging-in-Publication Data
Bond, Mary, 1942–
The new rules of posture : how to sit, stand, and move in the modern world / Mary Bond.
p. cm.
Includes bibliographical references and index.
ISBN-13: 978-1-59477-124-8 (pbk.)
ISBN-10: 1-59477-124-3 (pbk.)
1. Posture. 2. Rolfing. I. Title.
RA781.5.B66 2007
613.7'8—dc22
2006027435

Printed and bound in Canada by Transcontinental

10 9 8 7 6 5 4 3 2 1

Text design and layout by Priscilla Baker
This book was typeset in Sabon, with Copperplate, Shelley, and Agenda used as display typefaces

To send correspondence to the author of this book, mail a first-class letter to the author c/o Inner Traditions • Bear & Company, One Park Street, Rochester, VT 05767, and we will forward the communication.

CONTENTS

Foreword by Leon Chaitow, N.D., D.O. ix

Preface xi

Introduction: What Are the New Rules of Posture? 1

■

PART ONE: AWARENESS

1. Your Conscious Body 16
2. Your Body's Internet 34

■

PART TWO: STABILITY

3. The Root of Posture 54
4. Healthy Breathing 72
5. Core Connections 91

■

PART THREE: ORIENTATION

6. Your Heart's Messengers 114
7. Footprints 134
8. Facing the World 154

■

PART FOUR: MOTION

9. Healthy Walking 170
10. Articulate Living 195

■

Afterword: Explore the New Rules of Posture, Together 215

■

Appendix: Therapeutic Resources for Healthy Posture 216

Bibliography 220

Index 223

EXPLORATIONS AND PRACTICES

■

1. YOUR CONSCIOUS BODY

Your Neutral Breath 17
A Stressful Moment 21
Simple Pleasure 23
Walking Inventory 24
Your Best Foot 25
Heel Strike 26
Pelvic Mobility 27
Arm Swing 28
Spinal Mobility 29
Head and Neck 29
Stabilizing Actions 30

■

2. YOUR BODY'S INTERNET

Postural Sway 37
Fascial Continuity 39
Sacroiliac Rocking 45
Holistic Impact 48
Counterrotation of Pelvis and Chest 49
Curling and Arching 50

■

3. THE ROOT OF POSTURE

Pelvis Palpation 57
The Pelvic Floor Diamond 59
The Anal Triangle 59
Slouching 63
Supported Sitting 64
Bending Over 65
Perceptual Fine Tuning 66
Smart Reclining 70

4. HEALTHY BREATHING

Quiet Breathing 74
Active Breathing 75
Global Breathing Awareness 84
Breathing in Your Back 85
Inhaling Beauty 86
Exhaling Surrender 86
The Spaciousness and Weight of Breathing 87
Breathing in Gravity 87
Slowing Your Breath with Sound 89
Healthy Breathing, Healthy Posture 89

5. CORE CONNECTIONS

Activating Your TA through the Pelvic Floor 97
Activating Your TA from a Table Position 99
Activating Your TA Lying Down 101
A Shortcut to the Inner Corset 102
Flying Table 104
Bending Forward and Bending Down 107
Posture as Relationship 110

6. YOUR HEART'S MESSENGERS

A Tour of Your Shoulders 115
Closing Your Shoulders 116
Shoulder Expression 117
Leverage 117
Shoulder Blade Pulses 118
Handprints on the Wall 120
Serratus Shortcut 123
Seated Sphinx 123
Reaching 124
Wall Traction 126
First Aid for Your "Mouse Arm" 128
Sacred Touch, Living Touch 131
Two-way Touching 132
Lifting Something Heavy 133

7. FOOTPRINTS

Self-assessment of Your Feet 136
Your Foot's Dimple 138
Relaxing Your Arches 141

Footprints on the Wall 142
Opening Your Feet 142
Alternating Pressure between Forefoot and Heel 143
Rocking from Stance Foot to Walking Foot 143
Stepping into Your Whole Heel 144
Help for Bunions 145
Aligning Your Legs 147
Shifting Sands 149
Sitting to Standing 151
Pushing the Floor 151
Sacred Ground 152

8. FACING THE WORLD

Jaw and Tongue Tensions 158
Nose and Palate Tension 159
Jaw and Inner Ear 160
Distinguishing Cranium and Face 161
Narrow Focus and Open Focus 162
Releasing Eye Tension 164
Receptive Eyes 164
Welcoming the World 166

9. HEALTHY WALKING

Stop and Go 175
Wall Traction Enhanced 178
Flying Table Enhanced 180
Hip Rotation 184
Counterrotation 185
Pelvic Gyroscope 186
Seated Spine Spirals 187
Initiating a Step 189
One Step 190
One Step with Rotation 192
Forget About It 192

10. ARTICULATE LIVING

Body Parts Art 197
Acceleration 203
Your Best Walk 210
Your Worst Walk 211
Walking Your Way out of a Funk 211

FOREWORD

Although there are sometimes structural reasons that prevent balanced posture and good use of the body, most of us are guilty of misusing our body machinery due to habit. As with all habits, these postural ones seem to be such a large part of our make-up that change appears impossible, difficult, or unnecessary. What Mary Bond has succeeded in doing in this delightfully written text is to demystify the processes required for the creation of better body usage.

The fact that most visits to physicians involve pain as a major symptom, and that most pain problems relate to the muscles and joints, shows just how important better body usage is. The muscles and joints are the tissues that bear the strain—and end up complaining—when we misuse our bodies while sitting, standing, walking, lifting, driving the car, and performing the multiple movements, in a host of postures, that make life worth living in our work and in our leisure activities. Body usage—good and bad—also has a direct impact on how our inner world of communications (nervous system), circulation, digestion and other functions work (or don't work), and is also a representation of mood, feelings, and personality. In addition to healthy muscle and joint usage, *The New Rules of Posture* explains the importance of the wonderful connective web that invests and supports all other soft tissues: the fascia.

At its very simplest it is worth remembering that the musculoskeletal system is the largest energy user in the body by a large margin, and when we misuse it and waste energy we are also loading a burden of strain onto areas (whether feet, knees, pelvic joints, spine, or neck) that will ultimately demonstrate disapproval of being misused by becoming tired, painful, and dysfunctional. As our joints and muscles start to complain, we too may also find ourselves becoming tired, pained, and less functional.

Poor postural habits are, however, only part of the story. This book also contains an excellent exploration of breathing, another area of poor habit that has enormous implications in relation to well-being—both physical and emotional.

Mary Bond explains all this material in an uncomplicated, elegant style. Using examples and experiential exercises combined with science- and experience-based explanations of what needs to be done—and how to do it—she shows how to reverse the inevitable decline into pain and dysfunction that follows misusing what has been called the "primary machinery of life."

To change any habit—and poor posture and poor use are mainly habits—requires, as a starting point, understanding. The explanations given in this book set the scene for understanding, making possible the next stage of learning—how to use our bodies more efficiently and safely.

Therapists as well as anyone seeking relief from the pain that results from poor postural habits should explore this gem of a book and follow its advice.

Leon Chaitow, N.D., D.O.
Honorary Fellow, School of Integrated Health
University of Westminster, London

PREFACE

One of my students gave me the assignment to write this volume. I'd been helping her discover how to sit and stand in ways that reduced the effects of her job-related stress. She was impressed that the simple things I showed her could make such a difference in her comfort. "There ought to be a manual," she said, "an owner's manual for your body."

The New Rules of Posture is that manual. The rules are new because they differ from the old rules, which teach posture as body alignment that is unrelated to what we feel. These new rules apply to our whole experience of living in our bodies as we move in relationship to the world around us. They are holistic because they approach posture as the expression of both mind and body.

A significant contributor to the holistic view of the body was Ida Rolf, who, in the 1950s developed a technique she called Structural Integration. Rolf's unique contribution was to view the human stance as being in relationship with the pull of gravity. Structural Integration, better known by its nickname, Rolfing, manually releases physical tensions that prevent the balanced alignment we call good posture.

In 1969, as a dancer ever searching for more flexibility and balance, I found that Rolfing gave me what I wanted. It also introduced me to an intelligence within my body, an experience so profound that I abandoned the dance studio to train with Ida Rolf. What I could not know at the time was that sharing the experience of embodiment with others would become my life's mission.

People who have had firsthand experience with Structural Integration know that it is far more than a manual therapy. Rolfing is, in fact, a philosophy; it is an inquiry into the nature of human embodiment. My hope is that *The New Rules of Posture* can help channel Rolf's inquiry into a mainstream conversation.

Since Rolf's death in 1979, many people have furthered her theory and techniques. Three of these contributors have profoundly influenced my understanding of posture and movement. The model of walking presented in chapter 9 is based on the work of Gael Ohlgren and David Clark of the Rolf Institute. Hubert Godard of the University of Paris and the Rolf Institute has brought Rolf's ideas to life in a theory about the perceptual nature of the body's interaction with gravity. My emphasis on reeducating the body through training the senses stems from my study with Godard. If Rolf's ideas are the foundation of this book, Godard's are its keystone.

My thanks to Ruth Barnes, Caroline Lewis Burton, and Sally Sevey Fitt for their helpful advice, to Stephen P. Miller for the lovely artwork, to Susan Davidson and the staff of Healing Arts Press, and to Katherine Kirby, D.C., whose editing made all the difference.

INTRODUCTION

WHAT ARE THE NEW RULES OF POSTURE?

"Hi there," said the pretty checker as she reached across the counter to scan my purchases. In an instant her friendly smile dissolved. "Oh, man! I've got to get to the chiropractor." I watched as she twisted her torso this way and that, trying to relieve the pain without attracting too much attention, but she had mine. Why was an attractive 20-something complaining about her body to a customer? True, it was closing time, the end of a long day, but it was only Wednesday and the new Target had been open less than a week. Her nametag said Carmen. Maybe she was in a fender bender, I thought, and that's why she's looking for a doctor. But it was just as likely that the way she used her body had her tied in knots.

We are all sculptors and painters, and our material is our own flesh and blood and bones.

Henry David Thoreau

As a movement therapist, it's my job to correct the poor posture and poor movement habits that underlie my clients' complaints and symptoms. People often consult with me as a last resort when conventional medical approaches have failed to give them relief. Sometimes it takes months of gradual change for someone to transform her posture enough to eliminate pain, but sometimes there's a quick and easy fix. I wondered whether I might find just the right comment to set Carmen on the road to healthy posture.

If I was to say something helpful, I needed to hit the mark with my assessment and offer a solution that would work right away. Most people have little patience for complicated advice about body maintenance. I scanned her body, trying not to be obvious. After all, she hadn't really asked for my help.

I watched her moving behind the counter. As she reached for my change, folding inward at the waist as she must have done dozens of times that day, my own body signaled, "Ouch!" There it was, I felt sure: low back pain. Carmen was among the 85 percent of Americans who experience back pain sometime in their lives.

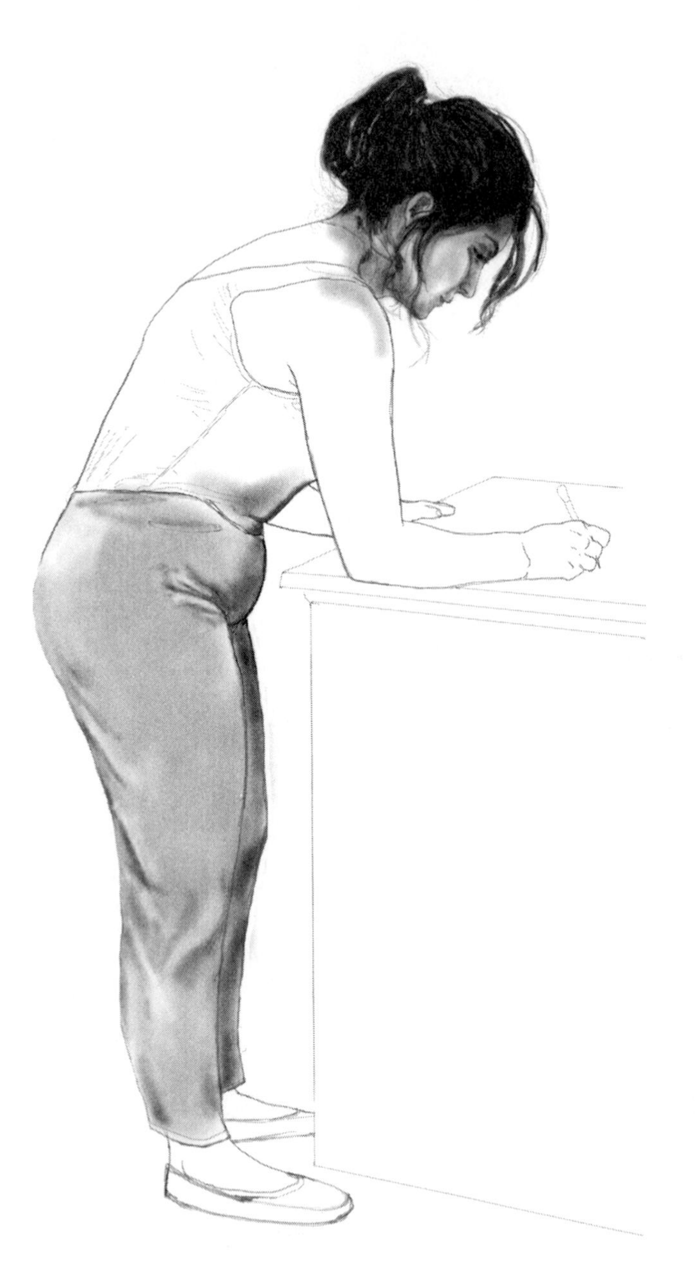

Fig. I.1. The way Carmen is bending over her work reveals poor abdominal support.

I ran down a mental list of potential ergonomic problems. The checker's workstation was a good height for her stature. It was neither so low that it forced her to stoop, nor so high that it made her hike up her shoulders to operate the cash register.

Next I considered the store's lighting. Although the fluorescent lights were overly bright, the checkout counter was near a window so there was plenty of natural light to counteract the overhead glare. Carmen wasn't squinting, but what about her eyesight? Sometimes eye strain makes people hunch over their work. Poor posture caused by poor vision can persist even after vision has been corrected. But Carmen's neck seemed free, with no trace of the forward-straining neck tension that accompanies faulty eyesight or hearing.

I glanced at the floor. Only a thin rubber mat protected the checker's feet from the concrete floor. Hard surfaces take a toll on the best of feet. Without good shoes, both feet and spine will suffer from long hours standing on such an unyielding surface, but Carmen's shoes looked sturdy. Barring foot problems that I couldn't see, the shoes seemed supportive enough.

Okay, then, what could I observe about the young woman's spine? As she stood there, Carmen's lower back looked balanced, neither overly straight nor overly curved. Could she freely bend and straighten it? When she leaned forward, I observed a smooth release of back muscles that let her vertebrae separate slightly as they must to allow forward bending. So, there was no problem with her flexibility. Her buttocks weren't tucking under either—a habit that might fix her lower back in a bent position that could make straightening up painful. It seemed that her spine was as adaptable as it looked.

Finally I saw both problem and solution. Carmen was stuck in a pattern I usually associated with women older than thirty, so it had taken me a while to notice. Camouflaged within the girl's tight jeans was a flaccid belly—not a fat belly, just an underactive one. I watched as she bent to retrieve a box of tissues that had fallen to the floor. She straightened and then reached down again for a shopping bag. Each time she bent down, her belly bulged forward. In healthy forward bending, the abdominal organs settle back into the abdominal cavity. Because Carmen's abdominal muscles were lax, her organs fell forward, putting unnecessary drag on her lower vertebrae. She desperately needed abdominal support.

If only I could show this woman how to engage what I call the inner corset. In my mind's eye, she grew statuesque. I imagined her jeans fitting better, her chest opening, her shoulders relaxing, and her back pain a distant memory. And, with better abdominal support, Carmen might unexpectedly benefit from improved digestion. Emotionally, she'd be better able to contain her "gut feelings" and have better boundaries in her relationships.

She'd bagged my purchases by now. It would take only minutes to explain. . . .

But it was closing time. Shoppers, many of them no doubt also wishing for a chiropractic adjustment, clamored in line behind me, hoping to get the kids to bed before ten. I handed Carmen my card. "I can help you with your back," I said as the customer behind me jostled into place. The checker gave me a blank look. "Have a good night," she said.

Your Posture Is Your Story

The book you're holding in your hands is my attempt to show you what I wanted to show Carmen: the relationship between your posture, your pain, your habits of movement, and your aging process. Our culture's assumption about getting older is that posture will deteriorate and the body will become a burden. If this is our belief, it is no wonder that we'd rather not think about caring for our bodies.

Perhaps you, like Carmen, are still in your twenties and not yet giving thought to growing older. Aging happens to us all, however, and knowing how to use your body well will make a huge difference in how you experience the process. Carmen, if she does not change her habitual way of doing things, will find herself at age fifty with hunched shoulders, a forward head, a thickened waist, and a protruding belly. She'll try to straighten up but will find that holding herself erect demands too much effort. Added to her back pain will be a host of other symptoms: headaches, a sore shoulder, digestive problems, and, although she won't like to talk about it, urinary incontinence. She'll find it hard to enjoy the kind of things she now loves to do, like salsa dancing on Friday nights.

Such a picture is not an unfamiliar one, but it does not have to be true once you understand how to manage your body in harmony with the principles set forth in this book. You can have a body that stands gracefully and moves effortlessly throughout life when you learn to use it the way it is designed to be used. It is never too soon, or too late, to create healthier posture.

Most people think about posture as the body's alignment or position when sitting or standing still. Good posture is commonly defined in terms of the contours of the upper body—the chest, shoulders, spine, and neck. Although people may be aware that balance over the feet has something to do with good posture, this usually is not what they consider first.

If this is your definition, I'd like to help you to expand it. I see posture not as how you hold your body when you're still but as how you carry it while you're moving. This distinction reveals posture to be a dynamic activity rather than a static attitude. Your posture is generated by your movement—by the way you carry yourself as you proceed through your life.

To determine whether your posture is healthy or not, I would want to see how you move, and I would consider the movement of your entire body, from soles to crown. Healthy posture is characterized by an easy grace, with movement flowing effortlessly between limbs and trunk. The movement of someone with unhealthy posture looks disconnected and labored.

How we carry our bodies evolved from how we were supported and regarded by other people from the time we were born. How Carmen bends over could derive from hundreds of experiences that have shaped her body usage. She was tall as a teenager, so perhaps her slouch was an attempt to be eye-to-eye with shorter boyfriends. It could have to do with not wanting to be a center of attention. She could feel imprisoned by her job or resentful about the way her life is going. Maybe the compression in her gut has to do with a baseball that knocked the wind out of her when she was fourteen. Whatever the source of her tensions, they have distorted her body to the extent that, at the ripe old age of twenty-two, her posture is creating pain.

Your posture emerges from your interactions with the world around you. It emerges out of how you orient yourself to the events of your life, how those events feel in your body, and how you move toward or away from the people or things involved. In time, your responses program the way you stand and move.

In addition to being shaped by your personal history, posture is also influenced by cultural and religious standards, by geographical features such as crowded streets or open terrain, by weather and clothing, and by media images that dictate what is attractive. Underlying all these relationships with the world is another more foundational one: your relationship with gravity.

Our bodies are inherently unstable because they are designed for mobility. The skeleton—basically an assemblage of struts, stilts, and levers—has hundreds of mobile joints. The muscles and other tissues that bind the skeleton together, and the organs contained within it, are nearly 70 percent water, making them even more mobile. The instability of this design renders our bodies plastic enough to adapt to the internal fluctuations of breathing, digestion, and other life processes as well as to the variety of positions we assume as we move about. However, without some means of securing such a mobile arrangement against gravity's downward pull, it would be impossible to take a single step. Gravity, as Sir Isaac Newton told us long ago, dictates falling.

For the most part, we do not fall because our bodies are programmed to negotiate with gravity. As we grow, creeping and crawling our way onto two legs, the nervous system coordinates our motions with increasing sophistication. As toddlers reaching out for a bright red ball, we pushed against the ground, first with knees and later with feet, as we struggled to outwit gravity and move towards our goal. Through trial and error, we learned to stabilize our bodies so we could control our limbs and move with purpose. Once walking, we then figured out how to run and play and work, always poised between falling and not falling.

We cannot separate posture from movement or activity from how we stabilize our bodies in order to act. How we stabilize ourselves determines our posture and the freedom, efficiency, and grace with which we move. The essence of posture, then, is the unique way in which each of us negotiates between moving and holding still in relationship to gravity.

Orienting and Stabilizing

We organize our posture in two ways: by orienting our body in space and by stabilizing it so we can move without falling.

Orienting is the process of knowing where you are before you move. If you're lost in the mountains, you orient yourself by looking for familiar landmarks. Upon waking from a dream, you orient yourself by recognizing the clock on the bedside table. With regard to your body, you orient yourself by sensing support from the ground and by being aware of the space surrounding your body. Although they are usually unconscious reactions, these sensory impressions let you feel secure enough to move. Your perceptions also help you automatically align your physical structure, centering it along a vertical line between earth and sky. In this way, your orienting perceptions help you resist gravity's demand.

For most of us, one of our orienting perceptions is less clear than the other. If the sensation of support from the ground is weak, we unconsciously feel insubstantial. We may brace ourselves with tension as a way of staying grounded, or we may literally gain weight to counteract a sense of being adrift.

On the other hand, if our awareness of the space surrounding our bodies is limited, we become too rooted to move expansively. By limiting our point of view, excessive grounding can keep us holding on to beliefs, jobs, or relationships long after it is time for us to move on. Whether we are overly grounded or not grounded enough, our faulty perceptions make us feel insecure, and we deal with this by unconsciously seeking stability in other ways.

Although orienting takes place through sensory perception of what is outside the body, stabilizing occurs through muscular activity within it. We stabilize our bodies by stiffening one part to give leverage to another part. For example, when you open a jar, one hand stabilizes the jar so the other can turn the lid. If the lid is stuck tight, you unconsciously stiffen muscles along one whole side of your body to help immobilize the jar. In a similar way, when you walk, the muscles of one leg contract to provide an instant of stability so your other leg can swing forward.

Our muscles wrap around our skeletons in layers, like layers of clothing. In general, the outer muscle layers produce the visible motions of the arms, legs, and trunk, while deeper muscles provide support for joints and internal organs. Contraction of these deep muscles lets us create the stability we need to control our actions.

If we are well oriented to our surroundings, we can stabilize ourselves in ways that allow our bodies to remain open and expressive. But if orientation is insufficient, we compensate by stabilizing too much. We contract our muscles in ways that diminish our dimensions, making our bodies shorter, narrower, or flatter, and effectively closing them. We do this by means of subtle contractions of muscles that lie in the deep layers of our bodies. These inward protective, stabilizing acts are as expressive as any outward gesture, like the traffic cop's outstretched hand that signals "stop."

Such internal closure compresses our joints and internal organs and limits our capacity to adapt to life's demands. By steeling ourselves in relation to events in the world around us, we build, little by little, poor movement habits and unhealthy posture.

We accumulate these habits of internal closure through our repeated attempts to stabilize our lives. Whenever we feel overwhelmed, we experience some degree of deficiency in our perception of the ground, our surroundings, or both. The resulting insecurity arouses a basic fear—the fear of falling. This, in turn, increases our need to stabilize our bodies.

Suppose you're interacting with an abusive boss. Without realizing it, you hold some part of your body still in order to manage your behavior during the confrontation. Tension in your jaw, throat, or shoulders keeps you from lashing out and losing your job. Tension in your hips or feet keeps you from storming out of the room. Similar tensions may arise when you deal with relatives' expectations of you or during a disagreement with a friend.

Pain also demands stabilization. When something hurts, we instinctively grasp the injured part with our hands. Striving to keep the wounded area as still as possible, we move the rest of the body around that still point. When something hurts intensely, we immobilize almost everything. People who are experiencing lower back pain move this way.

We also hold our bodies still in response to the dangers in our lives or to insults, memories, or even imagined events. Threats may have been physical or nonphysical. You could have been hit by a baseball, by a truck, or by harsh words. Whatever the circumstance, it was, or felt like it was, life-threatening at the time. When events spin out of control, most people respond by holding tight within the body's interior. This can be an attempt to protect vulnerable internal organs or, like a rabbit cornered by a coyote, to hold so still as to become invisible. Unlike a rabbit, which shakes itself and hops away when the threat has passed, humans tend to retain their internal tensions. The awkward movements of many people on city sidewalks are manifestations of such protective closure.

When threats are repeated, our protective responses become chronic tensions—often secret even from ourselves—held within the cores of our bodies. The responses become habitual because they worked: we survived. Although the initial danger has long past, we continue to experience a version of the original reaction whenever we experience stress. Even inconsequential stress—a broken fingernail, a traffic jam, a bad phone connection—evokes a remnant of emergency tension.

Slowly but surely, protective tensions erode our open orientation to earth and sky. Our plastic, mobile bodies become closed and solidified by the ways in which we stabilize ourselves. Excess stabilization shortens us as we age and, by reducing the range of motion of our joints, limits our enjoyment and expression of life. By overstabilizing, we fall, in slow motion, into gravity's embrace.

This book gives you tools for preventing or reversing this process.

Six Healthy Posture Zones

It will be evident by now that healing your posture cannot be a quick fix, although posture improvement programs usually promise just that. Conventional programs focus on reshaping your body's outer form. They teach you to align your body along a vertical line through your ears, shoulders, hips, and ankles—the line of gravity's pull—and to strengthen muscles to maintain that alignment. While it is true that most people hold their bodies behind gravity's axis, simply positioning the body more forward is merely a mechanical adjustment. It does nothing to change your perceptual relationship with gravity or the world around you. The activity of changing your perceptions is what makes changes in posture sustainable.

Your deeply ingrained orienting and stabilizing habits determine how readily you can sustain any outer adjustments to your posture. Take "shoulders back" for example. It is uncomfortable to hold this shoulder placement for long if tension within the body is drawing the torso down and forward. In a struggle between outer and inner, between shoulders and gut, the gut will always win. In addition to strengthening the shoulders to hold them back, we also need to practice the creation of new sensations within our bellies and chests. Healing posture entails more than just strengthening muscles to hold our bodies in alignment.

Through the perceptual approach presented in this book, you will realize that healthy posture is not an ideal shape toward which you must strive, or even something you must *do* differently with your body. Instead it is something different that you learn to *feel*. By approaching postural change from the inside out, the new rules of posture help you develop new sense memories for what feels balanced and stable. These sensations automatically bring your body into alignment with gravity. For most people, this means that their bodies will balance more forward over their feet. Their bodies will also lengthen and be taller.

This does not mean that fitness is irrelevant to your posture. Without strength and flexibility, you cannot maintain an adaptable relationship with gravity. If your only exercise is a click of the remote, you are more likely to trip over a curb or emotionally crumble under a snarled relationship than you would be if you took time for a daily walk or workout.

Exercise without body awareness, however, can actually make poor posture worse. By strengthening your muscles around a compressed infrastructure, you close your body more, solidifying your body's imbalances. By identifying and correcting specific tensions within your body, as this book will show you, you will add posture-enhancing benefits to any fitness program.

The New Rules of Posture helps you explore six regions of your body involved in creating open or closed stability, depending on how you use these regions. The posture zones include your breathing muscles, abdomen, pelvic floor, hands, feet, and head. The first three of these key areas are structures that contain your body's core and through which you stabilize yourself internally. The last three help you orient to and relate with the world. The six regions are connected anatomically, so activity—tension or release—in any one area always affects the others.

By learning the correct use of each posture zone, you build open stabilization within your body and open orientation to the world around you. As you work with the posture zones, you will identify tensions that close and compress your body. You will

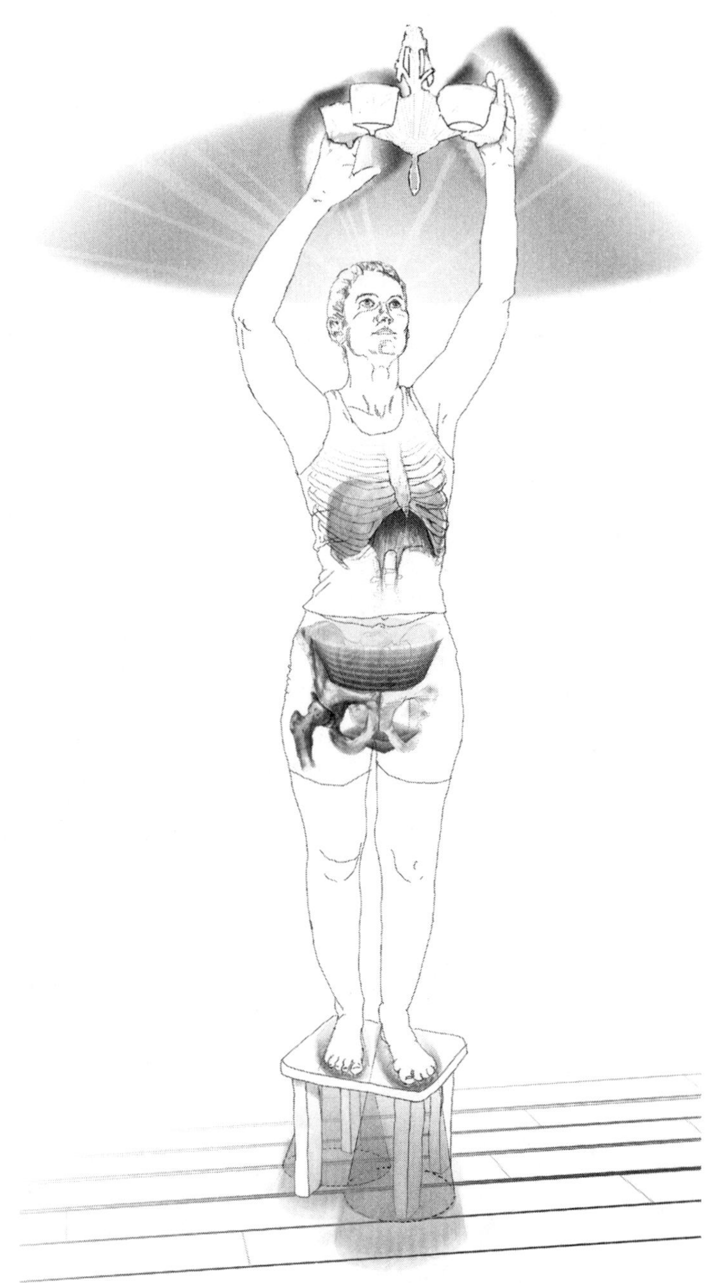

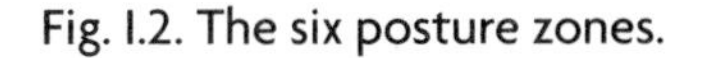

Fig. I.2. The six posture zones.

replace closing tensions with new sensations of stability and with new ways to orient yourself to situations and people. Gradually, you will exchange closure for an open stability that feels even more secure because it lets you move freely. Also, because posture is generated by movement, the way you move will change. In these ways, you will restore your body's natural alignment. Then, with gravity as a dynamic partner, you will raise your potential for grace, efficiency, and vitality.

This book coaches you through this process, and, like any good coach, it teaches you to coach yourself.

How to Use This Book

The New Rules of Posture is not a typical self-help book in that it does not offer a formula that works the same way for everyone. It can't, because each person's posture is the result of a complex set of habits blended together in a unique way. What the book does offer are principles of structure and movement that will help you learn how to best use your body. As you coach yourself through the accompanying exercises, you will bring your body into harmony with those principles.

The book is organized into four parts. Part 1, "Awareness" (chapters 1 and 2), readies you for the transformational work in the ensuing parts. In part 2, "Stability" (chapters 3–5), you will learn about ways to stabilize your body's core. Part 3, "Orientation" (chapters 6–8), explores the relationship between how you touch and perceive your environment and how you stabilize yourself and move. Every chapter includes explorations to increase your awareness, examples of simple anatomy that will help ground your awareness in physical reality, and tips on using your new awareness in daily life. Specific issues like lower back pain and repetitive stress injuries are also addressed. Part 4, "Motion" (chapters 9 and 10), draws everything together into a comprehensive experience of healthy posture in daily life. This includes walking and ways to incorporate principles of healthy posture into your fitness regime.

Approaching your posture from the inside out, you will not be trying to train your muscles into assuming an ideal shape. Instead, you will be developing sensations and perceptions that allow healthy posture to occur. This will involve a different style of exercise than what you may be used to.

The exercises in this book are of two types. Explorations are exercises that you will do once or twice to appreciate something about how your body works or could work. To do them, you'll need to put the book down, find a place where you will not be distracted, and devote several minutes to becoming more intimately acquainted with your body. Other exercises, called practices, involve more time and commitment. Although they do not require great effort, they do need your undivided attention. The practices are more like meditations than they are like conventional exercises and will not be effective if they are performed in a mechanical way. Your ability to focus on subtle body sensations will increase as you move through the book and as the practices increase in complexity.

Together, the explorations and practices will take you on a journey through the internal tensions that determine the outer shape of your posture. As you explore the subtlety of your tensions, you may encounter your body—and your self—in unexpected ways. You may discover tensions you didn't know you had and bring parts of your body that have lost awareness back to life.

For the journey, you need to bring along your curiosity and a spirit of adventure. Along the way, you will meet a cast of characters who, like Carmen, need help understanding their bodies. You'll watch as they transform their poor postures and eliminate pain through their commitment to body consciousness. The characters are composites of my students, and their stories were chosen to bring life to typical posture problems and solutions.

I suggest reading the book straight through once to get an overview of the program. This initial overview may be daunting in that you'll become aware of the many influences on your posture. Don't let that stop you. Then go back and explore the book, working through it one chapter at a time. Experience each chapter, do the work, and trust that healthy posture will evolve. Don't set out to keep track of everything at once. If you do, you'll use the part of your brain that is good at analyzing things but clumsy at coordinating your body. By making progress in each zone, your whole body improves because the posture zones are interconnected.

If paying attention to your body is new to you, pursuing the program can have its ups and downs. Some practices may seem confusing or so subtle that you'll wonder whether you're accomplishing anything. Be assured, as long as you keep paying attention, you will make progress. Keep traveling though the book, skipping any practices you don't understand. When you return to them later, they will make more sense. Coach yourself gently. Adopt the attributes of the best coaches: patience, persistence, and a sense of humor.

How much time you devote to developing healthy posture depends on you. If you can only spare fifteen minutes out of your day, begin with that. Even a few minutes of focused awareness will have a beneficial effect. Most of the practices can and should be incorporated into your daily living once you understand them. That means your posture practice can take place while you're taking a walk, making the bed, sitting at your desk, or working out at the gym.

In fact, the awareness you gain through working with this book will amplify the benefits you gain from any exercise. It will also improve your performance in any activity. Through the methods set forth here, I've watched golfers refine their swings, runners improve their times, and yoga practitioners find effortless balance. Lovers have even reported more satisfying lovemaking.

If you can, share your adventure in body awareness with a friend. New habits take hold better when they are witnessed by others. Better yet, form a group to explore the new rules of posture, using this book as your frame of reference. You'll find suggestions for doing this in the afterword.

How long it will take to feel improvement varies from person to person. As I said earlier, there's no quick fix for something so complex as posture. As long as you decide that healing your posture is important and make time for it, transformation will occur. The more you use your body as it is designed to be used, the better your posture will become and the better it will feel. Conversely, poor use invites deterioration. You can get better or you can get worse, but gravity will not allow you to stay the same. What this adds up to is that keeping your posture healthy is a lifelong endeavor. This book is your reference, your how-to manual, and your travel guide.

The new rules of posture, simply stated, are:

- Cultivate healthy posture through a process of self-study. You will need to create new sense memories for what feels balanced and stable through the means suggested in the following chapters.
- Remember that your posture is a dynamic activity, not a static position you can assume and then forget about. Your posture is the ongoing perceptual process by which you orient yourself to gravity and to your relationship with the people, objects, and events in your world.

Living in Your Body

Imagine yourself strolling though a pleasant neighborhood some sunny afternoon. You notice five-year-olds dancing through a sprinkler, their bodies like bobbing corks. Spines resilient and arms flying, the children hop, leap, squat, and jump without a trace of effort.

Further on, passing a Burger King, you see those same children ten years older, with their chests depressed, shoulders rounded, tails tucked under, and heads hanging. What intervening trauma, shame, peer pressure, fashion, rebellion, and failure of physical education have wrought such poor posture?

Ten years later (in Starbucks now), that posture manifests as occasional jaw pain; headaches; and neck, shoulder, or low back pain. With such intermittent complaints, most twenty-somethings plunge into their thirties, perhaps starting a fitness program, perhaps just getting by on youthful vigor. Creative in adorning their bodies, they have not yet been faced with responsibility for their bodies' well-being.

Long hours at ill-fitting workstations and worse-fitting car seats take their toll. In their forties, fifties, and later, protruding abdomens, dowager's humps, sciatica, and bunions get the better of these people and they look around for help. Doctors stand ready to suction, cut, and medicate, but the wiser and luckier of these people turn to yoga, alternative fitness programs like Pilates, and alternative healing methods including bodywork and movement therapy.

Carmen, we'll see, doesn't wait until her fifth decade to recognize her need for heathier posture.

PART ONE

AWARENESS

Tell me and I forget. Show me and I remember.
Involve me and I understand.

CHINESE PROVERB

1 YOUR CONSCIOUS BODY

The mysteries of the soul are revealed in the movements of the body.

MICHELANGELO

As you linger outside Starbucks one morning, your eye catches a movement a block away. The woman's walk has a familiar shape and rhythm, as familiar as a popular song you haven't heard in years. You crane your neck for a clearer view. While you can't make out the face, you know it has to be Mika, your neighbor down on Oak Street—when was it?—at least ten years ago.

She draws closer. It's Mika, all right. Her unique posture and movements gave her away.

The capacity to tune in to the rhythm, energy, and shape of someone else's movements let our ancient forebears discern friend from foe. Your empathic recognition of another person's movements tells you who is climbing the stairs—the UPS man or your brother—by the sound of his footsteps. You might even know the mood he's in, depending on how well you know your UPS man. Yet we rarely use our body-reading skill on ourselves. Most of us ignore our bodies except when they hurt or don't look or perform they way we want them to. The explorations in this chapter will help you tune into the rhythm, energy, shape, and mood of your own movements and identify ways in which you currently stabilize yourself in relation to gravity. The explorations involve two activities that are constantly shaping your posture.

Every day, we take up to 20,000 breaths and at least 10,000 steps. Walking and breathing are so ingrained in our behavior that most of us don't think of them as habits that might need changing. However, by walking and breathing as we do, we perpetuate our postural habits, good or bad. How we stabilize our bodies determines both our potential for healthy breathing and our freedom to walk with efficiency and grace. We'll first examine your usual ways of breathing and walking and then look at how stress influences both activities.

Neutral Breathing

The movements of respiration vary depending on what you happen to be doing. You breathe differently, for example, when you're sleeping than when you're washing the car. For the most part, breathing is automatic—it happens whether you think about it or not. However, you also have voluntary control over your breathing that enables you to sing, snorkel, or stifle a yawn. The moment you think about your breathing, you interrupt the involuntary flow of it, so the experiment that follows can only give you an approximate sense of your breathing. Nonetheless, by developing curiosity about your breathing, you'll begin to catch glimpses of your involuntary habits.

Exploration: Your Neutral Breath

If you're reading this book while lying on the couch, you should sit up to do this exploration. The act of breathing is different when you are lying down than it is when you are sitting, and for now, we want to assess your breathing in ordinary waking situations.

Observe your inhalation and exhalation for several moments. Be curious about it, as if it were a phenomenon you had never noticed before. In addition to sensations of air moving through your nasal passages, mouth, and throat, where else in your body can you feel the movement of your breathing? Close your eyes for deeper concentration and spend a minute observing the sensations of your breathing throughout your body. Then go on reading.

You may have felt your belly moving out and in, your ribs widening in circumference, your chest rising and falling, and possibly some movement of your shoulder blades—gliding away from each other or rising slightly as you inhale. You may also have had a sense of your whole body swelling slightly during the inhalation and then settling or shrinking on the exhalation—as if your skin surface got slightly bigger, then smaller with each breath cycle.

Because everything in your body is connected to everything else, you can sense the movement of your breathing in places distant from your lungs—in your wrists or ankles, for example. You'll learn about connective tissue, the medium through which this occurs, in chapter 2. If you weren't able to feel your breath that far afield at this time, don't worry. Just know that such awareness is possible.

To understand your breathing better, it will be helpful to take a short excursion into its related anatomy. After that you'll return to an examination of your neutral breathing and explore what happens to it under stressful circumstances.

Anatomy: Understanding Your Diaphragm

In normal breathing, your belly moves out when you inhale and recedes when you exhale. This movement happens because the diaphragm—your primary muscle of respiration—presses down on your abdominal organs when it contracts, pushing them forward. Because the diaphragm is cru-

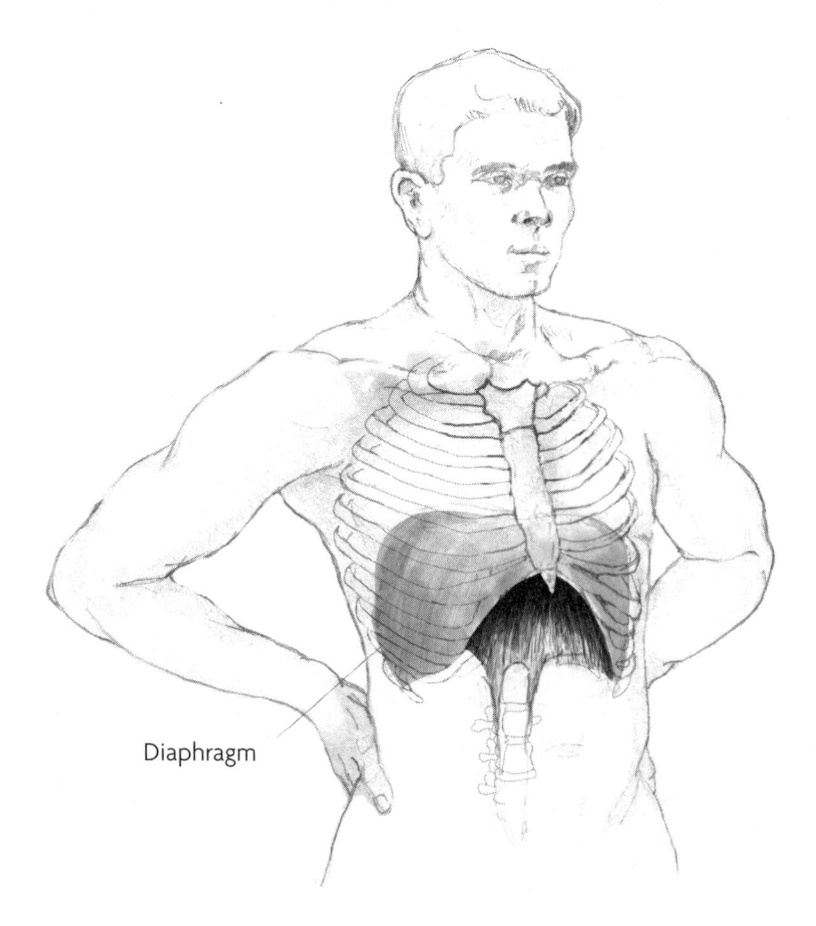

Fig. 1.1. The umbrella-shaped diaphragm is your primary breathing muscle.

cial to your posture, we will visit it many times throughout this book.

The diaphragm is a sheet of muscle about an eighth of an inch thick that is simultaneously the roof of your abdomen and the floor of your rib cage. It is one of the few places where muscle tissue lies across the body—roughly perpendicular to your vertical stance. The periphery of the diaphragm attaches all the way around the lower border of your ribs, from your spine in back to the lower end of your breastbone in front. The crown of its domed surface lies about halfway between the lower front ribs and the nipple line. Your lungs and heart rest above the diaphragm, and your liver, stomach, and intestines lie below it.

The diaphragm is attached to the connective tissue—called *pleura*—that wraps around your lungs. When your diaphragm contracts, flattening its dome onto your abdomen, its motion pulls down on your lungs. This stretching of the lungs creates a vacuum within the millions of tiny air sacs that compose lung tissue. Air rushes in through your breathing passages to fill the vacuum. Exhalation occurs when your diaphragm relaxes, pushing the air out by reassuming its dome shape. Breathing, then, is an automatic reaction, not something you have to make your body do.

Take a moment right now to visualize and feel the piston-like downward and upward motions of your diaphragm. Although the diaphragm descends only about an inch, it creates considerable pressure in the abdomen, something you've been aware of after eating a heavy meal. The movements of the diaphragm massage your intestinal organs, which assists in digestion.

The motion of the diaphragm has two important influences on posture. When you inhale, negative atmospheric pressure within your rib cage raises your chest. When you exhale, the mechanical action of your rising diaphragm helps keep your chest from collapsing. So, as long as there is nothing blocking the movement of your diaphragm, breathing contributes lift to your posture. As you will see, however, the diaphragm's action is easily disrupted by tensions elsewhere in your body.

OTHER MUSCLES OF RESPIRATION

Although the diaphragm is the main muscle used in inhalation, other muscles help the rib cage expand. Little muscles between the ribs cause the individual ribs to pivot at the joints where they meet the spine. You have probably felt your rib cage expanding or widening during inhalation, but the fact that individual ribs pivot may seem surprising. The motion of the ribs in back makes the front of the rib cage rise. The ribs also act as spacers between the vertebrae, so when they turn, they spread the vertebrae a tiny bit, lengthening the spine and helping it stay flexible.

To sense the motion of your ribs, place your hands on the back of your rib cage so your fingertips touch your spine and the heels of your hands and thumbs touch your side ribs. Let your fingers rest lightly. Because your fingertips and palms are very sensitive to sensation, you don't need to apply pressure to your rib cage to feel the motion of your breathing. In fact, the harder you press, the less you will feel. Visualize and sense the pivoting action of your ribs. Imagine the slats in a set of venetian blinds opening and closing.

Right at the intersection of ribs and spine, breathing and back tension are inextricably linked. Excessive tension in muscles along your spine prevents your ribs from pivoting; this, in turn, restricts your breathing. For healthy breathing, the ribs should move in relation to the spine; for the spine to be flexible, the breath must be unrestricted. To heal your spine, you must heal your breath, and vice versa. To heal your posture, you must heal both. Healthy breathing is one of your new rules of posture.

Another set of inhalation muscles lies along the sides of your neck and attaches to the first two ribs. When these muscles—the *scalenes*—contract, your upper ribs rise. Place your fingertips along the side of your lower neck, just above your collarbone. (Cross your right hand over to touch the left side of your neck, and vice versa.) Lightly rest your fingertips there without pressing. As you inhale, the contraction of the scalenes causes a subtle hardening of the tissue under your fingers.

The scalenes assist normal, unforced breathing but are more strongly activated if other breathing muscles are blocked. This could happen in any type of emergency. To feel it, take an "emergency breath"—a quick, sharp inhalation. Keep your fingers on your neck and you will feel the scalenes push up under your fingertips. If you have experienced some form of trauma, your scalenes may be chronically tight because overwhelming events interrupt the movement of the diaphragm and cause the scalenes to take over. Chronic tension in your belly also restricts the diaphragm and makes the scalenes overwork. Because these muscles must also work to bend and turn your neck, breathing restrictions and neck problems often go hand in hand.

In quiet breathing, exhalation occurs because your diaphragm relaxes. During times of activity or stress, your abdominal muscles assist the diaphragm in pushing the air out. These muscles, thin sheets of tissue that crisscross the abdomen like an old-fashioned girdle, compress your belly during

Sensing Subtlety

When you inhale, movement of the right and left sides of your diaphragm may not feel the same. This is due to your internal anatomy. On your right side, the diaphragm descends against your liver, the densest organ in your body. On the left, it presses down on your stomach, which, unless you've just eaten, is a hollow chamber. Take a few moments to feel the differing sensations on the two sides of your diaphragm. As you continue to work toward healthier posture, your capacity to notice subtle sensations within your body will grow.

forced exhalation, such as when you're running a marathon, laughing, or coughing. Try a little cough right now to feel how your abdominal muscles force your diaphragm upward into your rib cage.

Healthy muscle tone in the abdomen both supports the spine and assists with digestion and respiration. Constant upper abdominal tension, however, prevents the diaphragm from descending and blocks the natural lift of the chest that breathing should create. Such tension can develop by habitually tightening the stomach muscles in an attempt to appear thin, by performing abdominal exercises incorrectly, or through emotional constraint or digestive problems. As you'll see in chapter 5, the wrong kind of tension in your abdominal muscles contributes to poorer rather than better posture.

The Effect of Visualization

Your brain and body respond to imagined events with almost the same intensity as to real ones. Throughout this book, you will use imaginary situations to help you reveal or correct your habitual posture. Doing this will amplify your body awareness in actual situations.

Exploration: A Stressful Moment

In this exploration you'll discover what happens to your neutral breathing when you're under stress. Recall a mildly irritating incident that occurred recently—not a major trauma but a simple irritation, something like misplacing your keys or running out of cat food. Choose a situation that involved you alone, apart from a relationship with other people. Picture the situation in living color, hear the sounds of the incident, smell the smells, see your surroundings. Close your eyes and spend twenty seconds being present with your irritation. Then open your eyes and stretch the stressful feeling out of your body. Do this much before reading further.

People who have studied martial arts, underwater sports, singing, or meditation may have learned to regulate their breathing under stress, but for most people, stress makes breathing shallower, faster, and higher in the chest. Compared with neutral breathing, you probably felt your diaphragm moving less. You used your diaphragm to stabilize your body in response to the imagined stress—not a good use of your breathing muscle.

What else did you notice? Did your body as a whole feel bigger or smaller than before? More spacious or more compact? More or less pliable, fluid, or graceful? How about your perceptions? Were you more or less aware of your surroundings? For most of you, the stressful moment will have closed both body and mind.

Muscular Armor and the Fluid Body

In attempting to control stressful situations, we often contract our muscles in a way that blocks movement instead of creating it. Those muscles then become a kind of armor that prevents us from moving freely. Muscular armor limits the motion of your joints. When muscles on opposite sides of a joint contract at the same time, the joint in question stiffens. Under stress, this kind of antagonism can occur anywhere in the body, even in the body's internal core. To experience the sensation of having muscular armor, imagine yourself being in a great hurry. Remaining seated, think of all the things on your "to do" list. Imagine all of them being urgent. Hurry, hurry, hurry, but don't move a muscle. Then, sustaining that tension in your body, get up and walk around the room.

When you try to move with this kind of tension in your body, you must overcome the resistance of your own muscles. Your effort to resist the resistance makes it even harder to move. Because you're trying to move and not move at the same time, your potential for efficiency and grace plummets. You might have seen this in a tennis player who can't find her rhythm or heard it in a musician on an off night. You might have experienced it yourself if you've ever tried to cook dinner when you're angry or express an opinion when you're tongue-tied. Your muscular armor makes your movement feel heavy and awkward, as if you are wearing a body stocking that is a size too small. The tight garment seems to make the world grow small as well.

Muscular armoring is usually an attempt to feel safer and less vulnerable by making your body feel solid. However, that solidity interferes with your body's normal functioning by disrupting its essentially fluid nature. Your body's composition is 60 to 70 percent fluid, depending on your age and activity level. This includes your muscles, even though they become dense when contracted. Chronic muscular tension destroys your natural fluidness. When you've been on the receiving end of a great massage, your muscles regain fluidness and you get up from the table able to move more freely than before. Relaxation is the restoration of your body's fluidity.

The core of your body, where your internal organs are, is even more fluid than your muscles. Your abdominal cavity is like a soft aquarium densely populated with sea plants coiled around one another and constantly in gentle motion. Whenever stress compresses your joints and muscles, making your body more compact, there is literally less room for fluids to circulate and organs to float and glide. It's no wonder that stress-induced muscular armoring leads to digestive, circulatory, and other functional problems.

Some tension is inevitable. It is muscle contraction, after all, that enables us to get things done. The problem comes when we tense our muscles and keep them that way—when our embodiment of stress becomes so habitual that we are no longer aware of it or, worse, perceive it as normal.

When stress reactions turn into habits, your posture, your mobility, and how you perceive your choices all suffer. The habit of embodying stress is something you can change. You've taken the first step by noticing your body's reaction to a minor problem.

Exploration: Simple Pleasure

The following experiment should counteract the results of the previous one. Recall a pleasurable moment that involved you alone. Don't conjure up a feeling of bliss or ecstasy, just the memory of a simple pleasure: the smell of freshly baked cookies, a starry night, a hot bath, or the sound of welcome rain. Let your body revel in the sensations. Continue reading when you've completely embodied your simple pleasure.

You'll notice a difference in your breathing between this and the previous experiment. This time, breathing will have felt slower, lower in your body, and more complete. Other sensations typical of pleasure are a feeling of openness in your throat, softening of your facial features, and relaxation in your belly along with a sense of increase in the width across your shoulders and chest and the length of your neck and spine. Your hands and arms might have felt looser; your legs and hips more connected to the rest of your body. In general, your body probably felt more open, more fluid, and more vulnerable.

The feeling of vulnerability might take some getting used to, especially when you are around other people. Allowing your body its natural mobility can evoke feelings of exposure, embarrassment, and even shame. It can also foster your creativity and self-expression. Most of us learned to restrain the pleasure of "aliveness" when we were children, damping down our exuberance in order to sit still in school. Although studies suggest that students actually learn better when their bodies are allowed to move, our society continues to associate an expressive body with lack of discipline. Healing your posture might require that you revamp your relationship to cultural or religious views that demean the expression of sensual pleasure.

When you consciously access a pleasurable body memory, you induce more space in your joints, more lift in your spine, and more grace in every move you make. Simple pleasures, then, are resources for transforming your posture.

Recognizing Your Walk

Just as you might recognize a long-lost friend by the way she walks, you too are recognized by your walking posture, energy, rhythm, and use of space. Humans, even sedentary twenty-first century ones, walk more than we perform any other activity. The characteristics of our gaits are determined by many factors including cultural, religious, and family influences as well as accidents, illnesses, and other incidents of personal history. The walking explorations that follow may make you aware of some of these influences.

The explorations in this section will help you identify details of your walking style. They will give you a "before" picture against which to measure your progress as you move through this book. Do the explorations in a space large enough to move around without bumping into walls or furniture. Walk back and forth across the room at least once for each question. Make some notes about your impressions so you'll have a basis for comparison as you reexamine walking in later chapters. Better yet, get a few video clips of your "before" walk.

Walk in an ordinary way but with a sense of purpose, as if you're completing an errand. The goal can be a simple one, like walking across the room to pick up a magazine. Try to walk naturally and be observant at the same time. The questions draw attention to details of a variety of walking habits, so some questions will be more relevant than others to your body. Because there are many details to observe, you may wish to spread the explorations over several sessions. If a question makes no sense to you, skip over it. You can always review the inventory later for further insights.

Exploration: Walking Inventory

As you walk, does any region of your body feel more present and alive to you than the rest? Go with your first impression.

Your answer to this question indicates the area of your body that moves most freely. We get our sense of being alive through movement. Areas that feel less vibrant are tenser and less mobile. Areas of tension indicate that you are stabilizing that part unnecessarily. Don't cast this first impression in stone, however. Let's go on and look in more detail.

Imagine a divider between the right and left sides of your body. For the next minute, pay attention only to your right side as you continue walking.

Then spend a minute with your left side. Take note of any differences between the two.

Does one heel seem to strike the floor more emphatically than the other? Does one leg take a longer stride?

Does one arm swing farther or more strongly than the other?

Most people have some degree of side-to-side imbalance in their movement. Reasons for this include handedness, athletic training (a right-handed golfer, for example, swings the torso forcibly from right to left, over and over), repetitive work activities, compensation for injury (favoring an injured leg while it heals), congenital shortness of one of the leg bones, spinal curvature, or an emotional pattern, such as wincing away from negative attention.

Exploration: Your Best Foot

This exploration gives you more information about the balance between your sides. Stand comfortably as if you are waiting in line for movie tickets. Then take a step forward toward the ticket window. Notice which leg took the step, and which leg pushed off.

Stand at ease again, then step forward with the other foot. Chances are that not putting your "best foot" forward will feel oddly unfamiliar and uncoordinated.

What's actually important to notice is not the foot that steps out, but the other one. The side from which you push off is the side that you use to stabilize your body. You will tend to rest your weight on that leg whenever you assume a casual stance. The push-off leg will be stronger and may even be visibly more muscular. It also will be less adaptable and less free to move than the other leg. Frequently the leg on this side is the one that experiences chronic pain or tends to become injured.

When you've observed this about your legs, you'll notice that you subtly express the habit with every step. Your stronger leg drives your gait and gives it a faintly lopsided rhythm. The joints and muscles of your pelvis and spine accommodate to the habit of your legs. A strong leg preference can cause misalignment as far away as your jaw.

No one's body is perfectly symmetrical. If you observed a slight imbalance between your two sides, don't be overly concerned. A strong right or left imbalance, however, makes you susceptible to chronic pain or injury. If you feel this is true of you, it could be beneficial to consult a bodywork professional who specializes in postural realignment.*

*See the appendix for references for structural bodywork.

Exploration: Heel Strike

Now turn your attention to your feet. As you walk, consider the back and front portions of each foot: do you feel more pressure through your heels or in the balls of your feet?

Many people have little awareness of the front part of the foot. While it's natural for the heel to strike the ground before the rest of the foot, emphatic heel contact indicates that your heels are literally digging in for leverage to pull your body forward. Your body's relationship with gravity is out of balance. Instead of centering on your vertical axis, your body is held behind it. If you notice this feature in your walk, it is likely that muscles along the backs of your legs are short and tight. (To check, bend down to touch your toes.) These muscles have become like reins restraining your legs. When this is the case, muscles on the front of the legs and hips overwork, which makes them tight as well.

If this is your walking style, you probably have little sense of your body being propelled by your legs as they swing behind you. You might be aware of your legs as they step in front of you but not as they sweep behind or push off from your toes. Pushing off from the toes and buttocks of each alternating "back leg" supports the spine, lifts the chest, and imparts a sense of power, ease, and confidence. Practices throughout this book will develop your ability to walk in this manner.

Next, imagine a line down the middle of each foot from the center of your heel to your second toe. Do you sense yourself balancing more to the outside edges of your feet as you walk or to the inside? Either pattern indicates that your body receives inadequate support from your feet. An insecure relationship to the ground through your feet demands compensatory overstabilization elsewhere in your body. We'll address healthy use of your feet in chapter 7.

Exploration: Pelvic Mobility

Resume walking and bring your awareness to your hips. Ball-and-socket joints connect your thighbones to your pelvis. Imagine them working deep inside the flesh of your buttocks.

Chronic tension in your hips and pelvis can make it difficult to feel motion in this area. Such tension can be due to cultural beliefs about beauty and sexuality. Because our culture decrees that thin is beautiful, many women tighten the muscles around their hips in an attempt to appear slender. People who are overweight compress this region to mask sensations of jiggling fat in the thighs or belly. Because our culture construes pelvic motion as female, men develop hip tension to avoid appearing feminine. Hip tension can also be an attempt to conceal the potency of the pelvic region by holding it immobile. The less we move any part of our body, the less we feel it, to the extent that it can seem to be invisible. Any experience of sexual trauma increases the likelihood of hip and pelvic tension.

The function of the hip joints is to communicate motion between the spine and legs. As alternate legs swing, the pelvis and spine should rotate ever so slightly around the body's vertical axis. When hip tension blocks these movements, the whole body is affected.

Resume walking and notice your abdomen. Can you feel a subtle movement of your navel toward your forward-swinging leg? It's a tiny movement—your belly button shifts five to ten degrees at most. If you feel it, then your pelvis is rotating as it should.

Does your chest rotate in the opposite direction of your pelvis? When the spine, pelvis, legs, and arms are working in concert, walking involves successive counter-rotating motions around your body's central axis. If your rib cage presses down onto your abdomen, there is no room in your trunk for this motion to occur. Such compression of your body's core may reflect emotional tensions, digestive dysfunction, poor breathing habits, or all three.

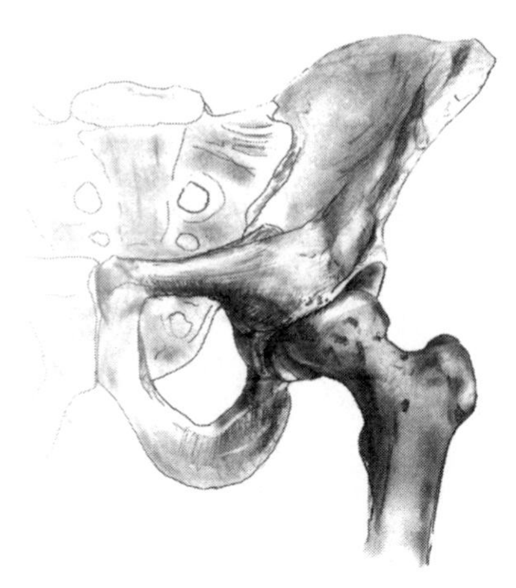

Fig. 1.2. The ball-and-socket design of the hip joints allows for smooth motion of the pelvis and legs in walking.

Exploration: Arm Swing

Next, tune in to the movements of your arms as you walk. Notice the swing of your forearm from your elbow. Feel your upper arm swinging from your shoulder joint. Try to sense a gliding motion of your shoulder blades against the back of your rib cage.

If elbow motion was the most obvious aspect of your arm swing, you are carrying too much tension in your upper arms, shoulder blades, or spine. There can be many reasons for this. Shoulder tension might reflect pain or instability in lower parts of the body: Someone might lift his shoulders in an attempt to take weight off of a painful back or knee or to compensate for unsupportive feet.

Shoulder tension is common in people who have sedentary lifestyles. Long hours of sitting with motion taking place mainly from the elbows down—as in computer occupations and driving—leave the shoulders little opportunity to move. Much of the tension of "hurry up and wait" that you explored several pages back probably occurred in your shoulders.

Just as pelvic and abdominal tension can be an attempt to disguise our shape or size, shoulder and chest tension can be a way of concealing the breasts. This habit is common among women who developed breasts early in puberty, who have large breasts, or who may have been subjected to inappropriate attention.

Often, though not always, tension around the shoulder blades is partnered with emotional restraint. Movements of the arms and shoulders reflect our connections with others: how we give, receive, and protect ourselves. With meaningful gestures like these, the shoulders act as gatekeepers for the heart. We all know how it feels to be given a "cold shoulder." We may also have felt the weight of shouldering too many responsibilities.

Whereas the vertical thrust of our legs and trunk organizes our stance and forward momentum, the movements of our arms define our social interactions. When fully spread, the arms make a horizontal gesture that expresses an open heart. The outstretched arms together with the vertical stance form the ancient symbol of the cross. The heart rests at the intersection of the arms and stance. When expressive movements of the arms are restrained, dysfunction cascades throughout the body. You can't walk powerfully or gracefully with your arms shackled. You can't breathe freely with your shoulders burdened.

Exploration: Spinal Mobility

Walking once more, notice the movement of your spine.

Many people sense little or no motion in their spines when they walk. Others notice only a side-to-side swaying pattern. There are two common versions of this. One is for the shoulders and chest to sway from side to side above the waist. The swaying helps the legs overcome the resistance of tension-restricted hip joints. In other words, the swaying compensates for lack of motion below. Actress Rosie O'Donnell often walks in this manner.

In the second common swaying pattern, the whole body rocks from one leg to the other, usually with the legs set somewhat far apart. This pattern is the stereotypical "jock" walk. It's a common compensation for back, hip, and core tension. By traveling on the edges of the body, the person avoids the sensation of movement through the center and expresses only the edges of himself. You'll see this gait in the early movies of Arnold Swarzenegger or on any football field.

When your spine is functioning well, it moves in three planes as you walk. One plane is the counter-rotation of the pelvis and rib cage described earlier. Another is a very slight sideways sway. The third is a subtle front-to-back undulation. When all three planes of movement occur simultaneously, the result is a spiraling motion, like the motion of water. You've seen this fluid multiplanar motion in wild animal documentaries, but it's rare to see it among your fellow pedestrians.

Whenever you are struck by the grace and sensuality of someone's movement, you are appreciating a healthy spine. Picture basketball legend Michael Jordan at the top of his game or actress Catherine Zeta-Jones. Such grace and sensuality depend on a capacity to stabilize the body without closing it with tension.

Exploration: Head and Neck

Notice what your head is doing as you walk in your usual way. Do your head and neck crane forward or hang downward? Is your chin set close to your throat, straightening your neck, or does your chin thrust forward, compressing the nape of your neck?

Our necks need support from the body structure below. Rounded shoulders and a compressed chest give the neck nothing to rest on. The neck must then hold itself up in addition to balancing the weight of an eight- to twelve-pound head.

Poor neck alignment often has to do with perception—with straining to see, hear, or understand. It can also reflect an attempt to block perception, as when we seek privacy by staring at the ground. Stress, especially stress that has to do with achieving goals, is another problem for our necks. We disorganize our necks whenever we get ahead of ourselves.

Neck tension affects the mobility of the entire spine. Because the ribs pivot at the spine as we breathe, neck tension can inhibit respiration and block the postural lift that healthy breathing creates. Vision or hearing problems also affect your posture. When you turn your neck to see or hear out of your better eye or ear, compensatory rotations occur down through your spine, pelvis, and legs as your body seeks to support the imbalance of your sensory organs. This means that a chronic sensory problem can affect your neck and end up causing strain in your hip or knee.

You Mean I Have to Learn to Walk All Over Again?

Although it may be disconcerting to face your postural patterns head-on, you know from experience that looking clearly at any problem is the first step toward solving it. Because you renew your posture—good or bad—with every step, embodying the new rules of posture will involve making changes in how you walk.

Learning to walk differently will take time. An infant needs three to six months to learn a new skill such as handling a spoon, sitting, or crawling. For adults, who must unlearn habitual movements along with learning new ones, and who, unlike infants, have other things to do besides exploring their bodies, it may take considerably longer. Real healing always takes time.

Exploration: Stabilizing Actions

The next exploration will help you observe how your relationships affect your body. While walking, you'll play out two scenes similar to those in which you contrasted the effects of stress and pleasure on your breathing.

In the first situation, an old friend, someone you feel 100 percent comfortable about meeting, is looking at you from across the room. Stand in a neutral position. See your friend. Walk toward her, letting your enthusiasm affect your body in an authentic way.

Notice how the experience affects your walking posture. It is typical to feel your arms swinging freely, a lift in your chest, an openness across your collar bones, lengthening in your throat and neck, softness in the muscles of your face, relaxation of your belly, fluid motion in your hips, energy in your legs and feet, and steadiness in your gaze.

Play it out a second time. Notice your rhythm, your emphasis and pacing. Notice how you take up space—how big your steps are, how generous your arm swing is.

For the second experiment, approach someone whom you admire and want to meet but whose regard for you is uncertain. Begin standing neutrally. See the person across the room. Then walk toward her.

How does this walk differ from the first? Notice your heel contact, pelvic motion, belly tension, arm swing, and eye level. Find words to describe the differences in your rhythm, spaciousness, and energy. Notice any sense of effort and where in your body you feel it. While the first exploration most likely improved your walking pattern, the second probably exaggerated its worst qualities.

In fact, your posture changed even before you began to walk. Did you notice? Think back to the moment when you were standing neutrally. Your posture changed the instant you saw each person. Try the experiment again if you're not sure. At the moment you saw your friend, you probably inhaled and smiled. Your body lifted and expanded, creating space in all your joints for ease of movement. When you walked, your feet were certain on the ground. This is how open stabilization feels.

In the second case, with the intimidating person, you may have noticed a subtle sense of closure within your body before you began to move. Maybe your belly tightened, your jaw clenched, or your buttocks tucked under. You might have noticed tension in your feet, as if you were standing on a very cold floor. Your head may have tilted down or to one side, altering your gaze. Overall, your body became slightly compressed.

Practical Body Consciousness

Your first reaction to a situation is to stabilize your body. Posture is the compound expression of your habitual stabilizing actions. In essence, your posture is your approach to life. How you perceive a relationship or a situation affects the ways in which you move, and how you move shapes your posture and your point of view. If your perception of the world is that people are generally well intentioned, the movements of your body will have more freedom than if you are unsure or anxious about your interactions with people. This applies to all the movements of your daily life—how you walk and stand, bend over and straighten up, reach for things and push them away, and how you sit, write, drive, and dance. Even how you breathe. The actions of your life mold your plastic body into its habitual shape.

Explorations in this chapter have highlighted the connection between your posture, your movement, and your emotions. The word *emotion* derives from Latin words meaning "from movement." The word suggests what our ancient forebears must have understood about the relationship between body and mind: that we experience physical sensations before we imbue them with meaning. What we call emotions come from our interpretations of our bodies' sensations of movement.

To develop sustainable improvement in your posture, you need awareness of the interface between your physical habits and your emotional connections to your world. This requires a different kind of body awareness than that used in a gym or fitness studio. Chapter by chapter, this book will help you refine your use of this awareness.

For now, remind yourself of the sensations you felt in the Stressful Moment and Simple Pleasure explorations. Experiment with substituting pleasurable sensations for stressful ones in common situations. This does not mean that you can turn disastrous circumstances into fun times but simply that you refuse to allow impatience or irritation to compress, immobilize, or numb your body. Waiting on hold for tech support is a perfect opportunity to try this. So is sitting at a traffic light or standing in a grocery checkout line. You'll find, too, that pleasurable body sensations foster positive thinking.

Tune in to your "pleasure body" before you engage in any fitness routine. Recall the fluid feeling of your body as you strode toward your friend. Tune in to those sensations while you walk, run, or swim or during your practice of dance, yoga, or Pilates. As you move through the book, you will gather more resources for handling the stress in your life without closing your posture. Cultivating your body's simple pleasure is a great way to begin.

In the next chapter, we will investigate the amazing system that connects everything in your body and shapes it for constraint or for freedom.

Meeting Mika

Always in a rush, Mika skims over the pavement as if gravity doesn't apply in her case. With her arms tight against her sides and her furrowed brow pitched forward, her body is streamlined for speed.

Her pace slows as she catches sight of you. Chin jutting forward, she squints, not trusting her eyesight. Then a wide grin accompanies a characteristic outward fling of her elbows, as if she'd fly across the dozen feet between you. Curiously, that gesture of flight seems to give her body substance. Her steps grow bigger, emphatic, and in no time you're clasped in a tight hug.

"Gotta fly," she says, after catching up for five minutes. You watch her body condense into its characteristic posture once again, thinking perhaps she'd reach her destinations in life just as fast and far more gracefully with the wide steps, free-swinging arms, and open chest of her "happy-to-see-you" stride.

Mika's posture derives from how she moves her body. By changing how she uses her body as she goes about her daily living she can change her posture. She needs simply to notice that how she moves makes a difference and decide that it is a difference worth cultivating.

2 YOUR BODY'S INTERNET

I sing the body electric.

WALT WHITMAN

Waiting for the light to change, mind on your shopping list, your gaze idly follows some pedestrians in the crosswalk. A woman, hunched over to wrestle with a shopping cart, calls out to a five-year-old, "Look where you're going, Rico! Don't run!"

She has your attention, if not her son's. In fact, when you start paying attention to your own body, you'll begin noticing pedestrian dance dramas everywhere.

A strapping teen, all shoelaces and baggy pants, struts along to an internal rap. For no apparent reason, he spins around and, with Jordanesque grace, swoops up the kid in one arm and cart in the other. "Rockie, you're an angel," calls the woman as she rushes across the street in his wake.

As the streetlight turns yellow, a bent, gray-haired man steps off the curb. You watch him, pursing your lips and thinking, "C'mon, come on, old boy." Cars from across the intersection inch forward as the fellow shuffles along. It's awful to be old, you think, as you watch the old man's struggle. Sighing, you release your grip on the steering wheel and reflect that maybe it's not just about age. After all, your dad, in his seventies, strides so vigorously across a fairway that you have to hustle to keep up.

Why do people move so differently? In the natural world, similar creatures move with similar pacing and rhythm. Except for soldiers marching, ensemble ballet dancing, and the strolling of new lovers, human movement tends to be idiosyncratic and disharmonious. The woman's bent-over bustling, the child's easy bounce, the teenager's careless verve, the old man's doddering—each has its individual combination of speed, rhythm, bodily shape, energy, and spatial range.

Many factors contribute to variations in human movement. Genetic inheritance, personal history, cultural background, nutrition, and environment are all involved. The circumstances of individual lives vary widely, and how our individual physiologies respond to life events varies even more. Posture and movement are commonly understood to involve complex activities of our skeletal, muscular, and nervous systems. Recent research has revealed connective tissue—which binds all the other systems together—to be a system in its own right. The connective tissue system is uniquely involved in the holistic approach of this book. This little understood aspect of the physiology of movement is the topic of this chapter.

Holism versus Mechanism

Most people address physical complaint to individual body parts: "My neck is too short." "My hips are too wide." "I can't reach my arm behind my back." "It hurts to bend over." In our neighborhood crosswalk, we can see Mrs. Garcia with her rounded shoulders and protruding stomach. Mr. Carlsen has a stiff spine and aching knees.

Pracitioners of conventional medicine and physical therapy view bodies as aggregations of damaged parts. They would give Mrs. Garcia a shoulder brace and teach her some abdominal strengthening exercises. For Mr. Carlsen, they would advise pain medication and, eventually, knee surgery. While the medical model of the body can be lifesaving, many chronic problems—as displayed by the two people in the crosswalk—would be better served by a holistic approach. Unfortunately, conventional medicine's endorsement of a mechanistic view of the body infuses our culture, influencing the way we regard and treat our bodies.

Among our bodies' many complex and intricately interacting systems, the connective tissue system pervades and provides structure for all the rest. Like the global electronic internet, it is a communication network that can connect any part to all the others. A short investigation of the connective tissue will make it clear why healing posture involves more than repositioning an offending body part.

Body of Water

We know that life began in the oceans. Over many eons, organic compounds derived from seawater developed into proteins. Some of these proteins formed a watery membrane that allowed evolving life forms to be contained and sustainable. This membrane was a primitive form of connective tissue. Collections of primitive cells gradually developed separate functions and, hundreds of millions of years later, evolved into primordial sea creatures. These creatures moved easily through water, but their spiraling, wavelike motions were not suitable for life on land. It took eons more for their soft, fluid bodies to evolve more solid tissues like bone and ligaments that let them move on land, where the effects of gravity are more strongly felt.

Human bodies are an incarnation of life's transition from water to land. Our skin and connective tissues form containers for the saltwater that still infuses all our tissues and cells. Our bones make us operational on land, able to walk and gesticulate, work and play. However, within our container of skin we are essentially aquatic.

Because most people unconsciously conceive of their bodies as solid, it can be surprising to know that our bodies' composition is approximately 70 percent water. Understanding this can give us a new perspective on transforming our posture because it makes it clear that our bodies are not dense and immutable.

Engineered for Motion

The conventional ideal of body alignment places body masses atop one another like a stack of blocks, lining them up so that gravity's axis runs through their centers and relying on the bony skeleton to sustain their weight. The problem with this model is that a stack of blocks doesn't move.

For a model that is more in accord with the fluid nature of the body, we borrow from the insights of engineering visionary Buckminster Fuller. He is famous for inventing the geodesic dome—the lightest, strongest, and most cost-effective shelter yet devised. Using pliable materials, Fuller used tension rather than compression to sustain his structures. He called his design system tensegrity.

If we apply Fuller's model to our bodies, we can see that it is the tensional force of our softer tissues that keeps us erect, not the compressional strength of our bones. Floating within a sea of fluid tissues, bones are internal spacers for the body rather than beams that resist compression. The length and tension of connective tissue adapts to the changing orientation of the bones and distributes gravitational forces through our bodies as we move.

Maintaining our upright stance is a process of perpetual motion. There is no such thing as standing still, or even sitting still, because the structural design of the body is inherently unstable. In the first place, the larger masses of the body are poised high above the narrow base of support provided by the feet. Second, the body's framework—the bony skeleton—is segmented, and the rounded edges of the interfaces between neighboring bones configure our joints for mobility rather than stability.

Without its guy wires of soft tissues, an upright skeleton, no matter how perfectly aligned, would quickly collapse into a heap. You have experienced this tendency at the end of a long day when your body crumples onto the couch. Although we sometimes think we are standing still, our nerves and muscles are making hundreds of tiny adjustments per second to orient our unstable frames against the pull of gravity. In the following exploration you can experience how this feels.

Exploration: Postural Sway

Stand with your legs slightly apart and your weight evenly distributed over both feet. If your usual stance is broad—with your feet set wider than your shoulders—make your stance slightly narrower than usual. Let your arms hang comfortably at your sides. Forget about maintaining good posture (we haven't gotten to that part yet), and simply stand in a comfortable, ordinary way. Close your eyes. If keeping them closed is uncomfortable, do the exploration with eyes open. Having closed eyes simply makes the sensations easier to perceive.

With your eyes closed, you will sense your body swaying slightly. Visualize your skeleton floating within the sea of your softer tissues. Experience the play of tensions through your ankles, knees, hips, and spine as your body negotiates its balance with gravity. Observe your movement for a minute or so, without trying to resist or control it.

You may sense a change of pressure through the soles of your feet or feel your torso swaying like the upper branches of a tree. The movement may seem random or it may repeat itself in an obvious pattern. If you are unable to perceive the motion, try standing on a slightly unstable surface such as a couch cushion or folded blanket.

What you are experiencing is known as postural sway. Everyone sways a little when they are standing. Military personnel at attention prevent the sway by contracting their muscles. Quirks in your sway pattern indicate imbalances in your posture. Let's say, for example, that you noticed yourself moving more strongly to the left than to the right. This could indicate that you have a habit of balancing yourself slightly to the left of center and could predict compensatory tensions in your left leg, left hip, and the left side of the spine. Stabilizing yourself left of center—or right, forward, or back of it—creates shortening and thickening of your connective tissue on that side.

THE ORGAN OF POSTURE

"Connective tissue" is a blanket term for all the tissues that separate, contain, and connect everything else in the body. Although Western anatomists have been studying the body for at least two thousand years, it was not until the twentieth century that connective tissue became a focus of study. Previously, anatomists removed it to reveal the muscles, nerves, and organs underneath. Even now, few anatomy books portray connective tissue. Yet this substance is every bit as vital as the reproductive, digestive, or other systems of our bodies.

Connective tissue is composed of a viscous matrix, also called "ground substance," that can be more fluid or more solid, depending on the demands placed on it. Protein fibers contribute structure to the ground substance, like the veins you see in the leaves of plants. When denser connective tissue is needed—to close a wound, for example—special cells within the ground substance produce extra fibers. A scar is fibrous connective tissue that forms to stabilize and protect an injured area.

Connective tissue has different names depending on its location and function. *Ligaments* are the fibrous connective tissues that connect bone to bone. *Tendons* connect muscle to bone. The delicate membranes that envelop your brain and spinal chord are connective tissues called *meninges*. Bone is a highly mineralized form of connective tissue. The tubing around nerves and blood vessels is made of connective tissue, as are the sheaths around your organs and muscles. This latter type of connective tissue is known as *fascia*.

Fascia does not merely envelop tissues; it permeates them, dividing the liver and brain into lobes and the heart into chambers. At the microscopic level, fascia forms discrete containers for every cell. If you liken the membrane around an orange segment to the fascia enveloping a muscle, then the thin film that separates sticky particles of orange can be likened to your microscopic cellular membranes.

Our bodies, then, contain a three-dimensional web of fascia with pockets and tubes for our various organs and muscles and with microscopic compartments for every cell. Connective tissues are everywhere; in fact, they make up about 20 percent of the body's weight. Anatomists have determined that were they to remove all other tissues from a body—liver, lung, brain, muscle, blood, fat, nerve, and so on—they would be left with a recognizable human form made of connective tissue.*

Adjacent fascial envelopes form continuous sheets that both separate neighboring muscles and connect distant regions of the body. The fascia along the crown of your head, for example, is part of an overlapping series of fascial connections that travels down the back of your body into the soles of your feet. You can experience your fascial continuity from head to toe with the following experiment. To do it you'll need a tennis ball and bare feet.

Exploration: Fascial Continuity

Stand up and bend over as if to touch your toes. Relax your neck so your head can hang down. Don't force the stretch—just notice how far you can easily go. Return to a standing position.

Now massage one of your feet by pressing it on the ball and very slowly rolling the ball across your sole. Include your heel and toes in the massage. You will be stretching the dense fascia along the sole of your foot and, because that is commonly tight, you may experience some discomfort. Spend about one minute doing this. Then remove the ball. Repeat the original forward bend, noting any difference in how it feels. Do this much before reading on.

You will feel that one side of your body—the side of the massaged foot—can now stretch farther toward the floor. Because the fascial fabric is continuous, crown to sole, stretching any part of it affects the whole. Be sure to massage the other foot so you'll be balanced before you sit down again.

The fascial track along the back of your body is only one of many pathways through the body's fascial "internet." A more central passage runs from the inner arch of the foot, up the inner thighs, through the pelvic floor, and along the inner surface of the spine behind your intestines. It includes your diaphragm and the

*Thomas Myers, *Anatomy Trains* (Edinburgh: Churchill Livingstone, 2001), 23–29.

fascia encompassing your heart, and passes up through the throat into the jaw and skull. Connecting paths run out the arms to the hands. The six healthy posture zones are united by this deep fascial passageway.

Connective Tissue Communication

Connective tissues provide a communication network that is distinct from our bodies' other means of communication, the endocrine and nervous systems. Because the ground substance of connective tissue has a liquid crystalline structure, it conducts bioelectric energy. Both compression and stretching send minute currents through the fascia, and these currents signal changes in its state. Maintaining a habitually closed posture induces fascia to produce more fiber. This is how poor posture becomes chronic.

Scientists have only just begun to understand how connective tissue works as an integrated system. Research suggests that the meridian pathways of Chinese medicine are energetic currents operating through planes of fascia.* Other studies indicate that fascia contains muscle cells similar to those that line the digestive tract.† These cells are responsive to the part of your nervous system that monitors unconscious functioning—further suggestion that our "organ of posture" is also an organ of communication.

Think back to the exercise in chapter 1 when you were invited to sense the effects of breathing in your ankles. Now that you understand more about the nature of connective tissue, that notion should seem less fantastic. The fascia of your diaphragm and lungs is connected with fascial sheets that lie along the inside surface of your spine and descend through your pelvis and groin. This fascia in turn is continuous with tracks that run down your inner legs to your feet. When, during inhalation, the descent of your diaphragm pulls down on the fascia around your lungs, it sends bioelectric signals all the way to your ankles. Try the breathing exploration from chapter 1 again. Sense the motion of your breathing in your ankles.

Fascia shrinks and toughens in response to any kind of stress: physical, environmental, or psychological. When your posture closes for an extended period, pressure through the crystalline ground substance signals special cells within your fascia to produce more fiber. This causes overlapping fascial sheaths to adhere to one another. The knots we feel in our muscles when we are tense result when adjacent layers of fascia stick together. Chronic tension in the upper shoulders, for example, causes fascia around the involved muscles to form adhesions that make it difficult to stretch out

*Helene M. Langevin and Jason A. Yandow, "Relationship of Acupuncture Points and Meridians to Connective Tissue Planes," *The New Anatomist* 269 (2002): 257–65.

†Robert Schleip, "Fascial Plasticity—A New Neurobiological Explanation," *Journal of Bodywork and Movement Therapies* 7 (2003): 104–116.

Structural Integration

Conventional therapeutic approaches to postural improvement are usually of limited effectiveness in dealing with strong fascial adhesions. Stretching programs are too general to address the unique tensions that produce individual postures. Strength-building programs often overlay an imbalanced frame with muscular bulk that actually worsens posture.

Structural Integration, developed in the 1950s by Ida Rolf, is a manual therapy that restores postural balance by releasing connective tissue adhesions. Rolf, in fact, was the first to recognize fascia as the "organ of posture." The slow, penetrating pressure of this style of bodywork takes advantage of the unique property of fascia to soften when steady pressure is applied to it. There have been various conjectures as to how manual pressure causes fascia to change its state. Current research suggests a combination of mechanical, biochemical, and neurological responses.*

Structural Integration therapists—sometimes known as Rolfers—are trained to perceive the holistic effects of each local intervention and to adapt the depth and pace of their touch to the client's developing body awareness. This prevents the process from being intensely painful. For readers who feel they need more than self-help, a series of Structural Integration treatments can augment the processes suggested in this book.†

*Robert Schleip, "Fascial Plasticity—A New Neurobiological Explanation," *Journal of Bodywork and Movement Therapies* 7 (2003): 11–19.

†The appendix of this book lists contact information for Structural Integration practitioners.

the tension. In a more extreme case, a buttress of fascia at the juncture of the neck and trunk forms to stabilize the exaggerated upper spine curvature known as dowager's hump.

In this, the fascia is only doing its job—stabilizing your posture—so you don't have to keep firing nerves and activating muscles to maintain the way you're standing or sitting. Instead, your connective tissue holds you in place as if with Velcro. Over time, the greater proportion of fiber within the ground substance slows metabolic exchanges and leads to the chronic stiffness commonly experienced as aging.

Because the fascial internet connects all body regions, adhesions in one place can create strain in distant areas. A stiff knee can derive from restricted fascial organization in a foot or hip, from adhesions around digestive organs, or even from imbalanced head position due to hearing loss in one ear. Any immobilized region tugs on distant strands of the holistic fabric, distorting the entire organ of posture.

The painful condition known as carpal tunnel syndrome occurs because nerves and blood vessels are caught between fascial adhesions of the forearm and wrist muscles. Hand pain can also be caused by fascial adhesion in the scalene muscles of the neck which compresses nerves that affect the arms. In either case, hand pain is a consequence of poor overall posture. Faulty sitting position, poor breathing, and insufficient abdominal tone all have bearing on fascial tensions through the shoulders and arms.

When fascia is healthy, it forms silky sheaths around our muscles, bones, joints, and organs. The smooth casings allow neighboring structures to glide across one another as we breathe and move, assisting healthy functioning.

One way in which healthy gliding of fascia can be blocked is through tension in our bodies' horizontal structures. Most of our muscles and their enveloping fascias run up and down along the skeleton, but in several important regions, muscles and fascia travel through the body from front to back and side to side. The parachute-shaped diaphragm, introduced in chapter 1, is an example. It rests horizontally, on a plane that is roughly perpendicular to the body's vertical axis. The floor of the pelvis and the floor of the mouth are also examples of horizontally oriented structures. The way we use our hands and feet puts them into this category as well.

Our vertically arranged muscles enable us to move, while the horizontal ones support our internal organs and help us manage our interactions with our environment. The crosswise muscles are the sites of our most interior motions of protection. They constrict whenever we hunker down under pressure. You can picture these crosswise tissues as valves located along your body's vertical axis. When tension causes a valve to close, it blocks gravity's clear path through your body. If tension closes your diaphragm, pelvic floor, or any other horizontal structure, your body compresses at that location. Such tension often spreads through the deep fascial layers, closing other horizontal structures as well. Such closure distorts both posture and movement. Habitual closure in these regions prevents you from sustaining good posture even when you try. The posture zones described in this book are all related to horizontally oriented fascial structures.

If you have poor posture, you know that your attempts to "straighten up" don't last for long. Your muscles are prisoners of their fascial envelopes. Unless fascial planes can freely glide across one another, the function of anything contained within those planes is restricted to some degree, keeping posture and habits of movement fixed.

When not prevented by postural closure, the adaptive gliding of neighboring fascial sheaths facilitates the integration of movement that we perceive as ease, sensuousness, and efficiency. Restricted fascia affects muscles so that movement looks and feels awkward. The spine, arms, and legs articulate freely only if their holistic fabric can adapt to the body's moment-by-moment relationship with gravity. When you admire the grace of Michael Jordan, Mikhail Baryshnikov, or Catherine Zeta-Jones, you are admiring more than muscular coordination; you are admiring a healthy connective tissue system.

Articulate Living

The concept of articulation is usually associated with verbal communication. When a speaker is articulate, she expresses herself easily and clearly through words, connecting them into meaningful ideas. Bodies are articulate when they are able to make efficient, graceful, and meaningful sequences of movements. This is what we admire in athletes, dancers, or actors.

In anatomical terminology, *articulation* is another word for "joint," the place where one bone moves in relation to another. It also means the way in which the parts of a joint work together. When overlapping fascial envelopes are free to glide across one another, they, too, are articulated. Ideally, every structure in the body should articulate freely in relation to its neighbors. Our organs, blood vessels, nerves, and muscles should glide fluently within their beds of connective tissue, and our hundreds of joints should all have free play. However, when adhesion reduces articulation, movement becomes jerky.

The articulate bodies of actors such as Cate Blanchett, Johnny Depp, or Anthony Hopkins enable them to assume a wide variety of roles. Their bodies' adaptability makes them versatile. By contrast, if an actor is more buff (consider The Rock), he will not be able to move his joints as freely and will give a less subtle performance. Articulate physicality also separates the elite athlete from the weekend warrior (Tiger Woods from Uncle Fred), and it separates the noble elder (such as Morgan Freeman) from the stooped senior citizen in the crosswalk. When bodies are not articulate, people look and feel old.

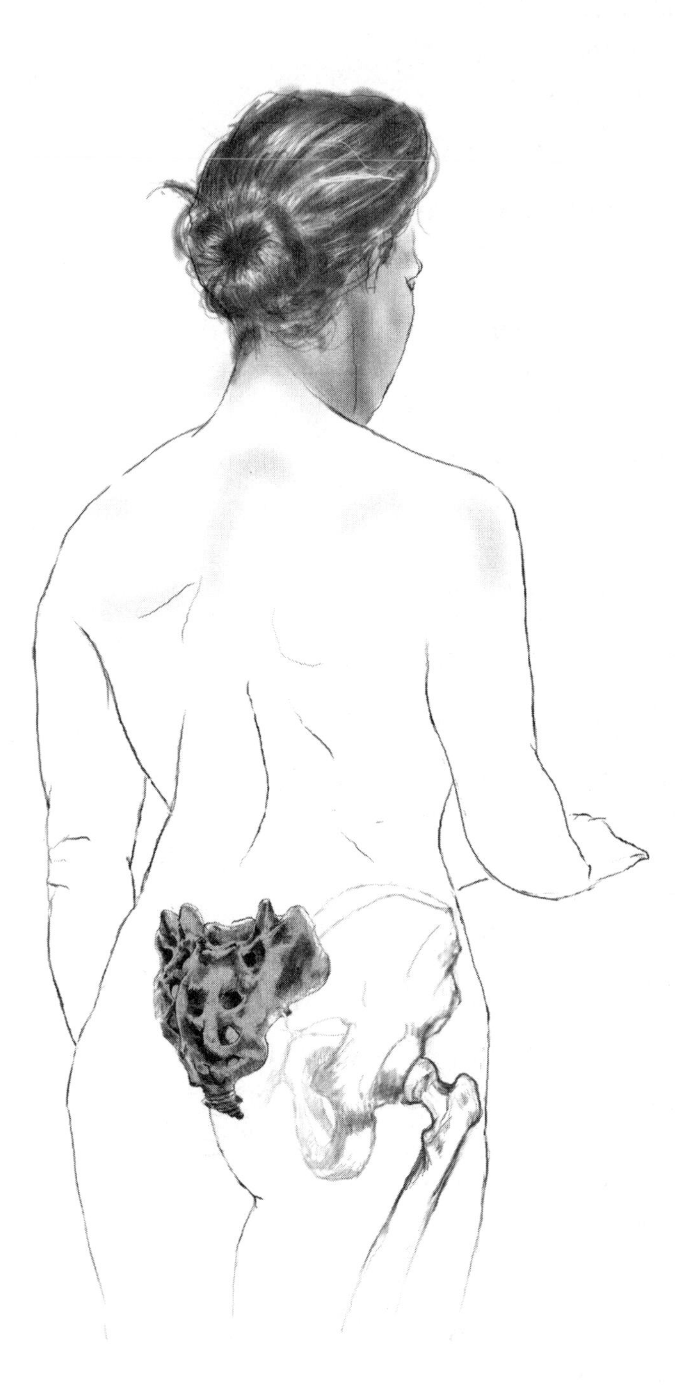

Fig. 2.1. Your sacrum is the base of your spine.

Although most of us do not aspire to elite performance, the comfort and elegance of our daily living depends on our bodies' capacities for motion. When joints and fascia are stiff, the nervous system cannot coordinate movement in ways that are fluid and efficient.

Exercises throughout this book are designed to increase your body's capacity for articulation. By keeping your connective tissues pliable, you not only improve your posture but also contribute to your overall health. Restoring articulation to your spine, for example, fosters healthy function of your digestive organs by helping the nerves and blood vessels that supply these organs to glide freely within their beds of fascia. The exercises that follow help you begin to restore articulation in your pelvis and spine.

Understanding Your Sacroiliac Joints

In this section, you will examine the articulation between the large triangular-shaped bone at the base of your spine, the *sacrum,* and the two pelvic bones on either side of it, the *ilia.*

To clarify the examination, we'll first take a brief tour of the anatomy involved. Look in a mirror at your lower back. You'll see two dimples above your buttocks on either side of your spine. The top of your sacrum lies between these two indentations. Standing in a neutral position, reach back and touch the dimples with the third fingers of each hand. Then slide your fingers diagonally downward and together to meet just above your tailbone *(coccyx)*. You have just outlined your sacrum. The sacrum is the base of your spine and is a sizable bone—about half an inch thick at its top. Directly in front of it lie your rectum and uterus or prostate.

Next, locate your ilia. Again place your third

fingers on the dimples and stretch the webbing of your thumbs forward across the top edge of each ilium just below your waistline. Then, slide your thumbs forward along the crest until you reach a drop-off point. Keep your thumbs there and let the rest of your fingers slide forward and down along the sides of your buttocks. Spread your fingers wide. Your hands are now covering the two fan-shaped ilia.

The joints between the sacrum and the two ilia (right and left *sacroiliac joints*, or SI joints) are shaped to fit together like two shallow spoons. The rounded surfaces on the sacrum face outward and fit neatly into the hollows on the adjoining ilia.

The shape of the sacroiliac joints allows movement in an area that most people assume to be immobile. In fact, the sacroiliac joints are elastic and flexible enough for each ilium to glide three to four millimeters forward and back across the sacrum. Although this is only a minute amount of motion, its presence or absence affects the movement of the entire body. In healthy walking, the two ilia should rotate opposite one another in concert with the actions of the legs. That is, as one ilium tips ever so slightly forward, the other tips back. Between the ilia, the sacrum nods slightly side to side.

In the following experiment, you will assess your own sacroiliac mobility. Sit upright on a chair without leaning against the backrest. Slide your fingers under your buttocks to locate your right and left "sit bones." Then release your fingers and sit with awareness of these bones beneath you.

Turn your spine to look over your right shoulder as if you are greeting friends being seated at a table behind you in a restaurant. Notice how your right sit bone has slid back a little bit, while the left sit bone has tipped forward. The phenomenon reverses when you turn to the opposite direction.

If you were able to feel your spine turning all the way down to your sit bones, then your sacroiliac joints were articulating. If you felt yourself turning above the waist or only in your neck, then your sacroiliac joints are stiff. The joints themselves are moveable but can be restricted by muscular tension around your pelvis and hip joints.

Practice: Sacroiliac Rocking

This practice will help you restore the sacroiliac mobility that you need for healthy posture and walking. Walk around a bit before you begin to give yourself a fresh "before" impression of your body. Then lie on your back on an exercise mat or carpeted floor. Rest your arms wherever they are comfortable. Position your head

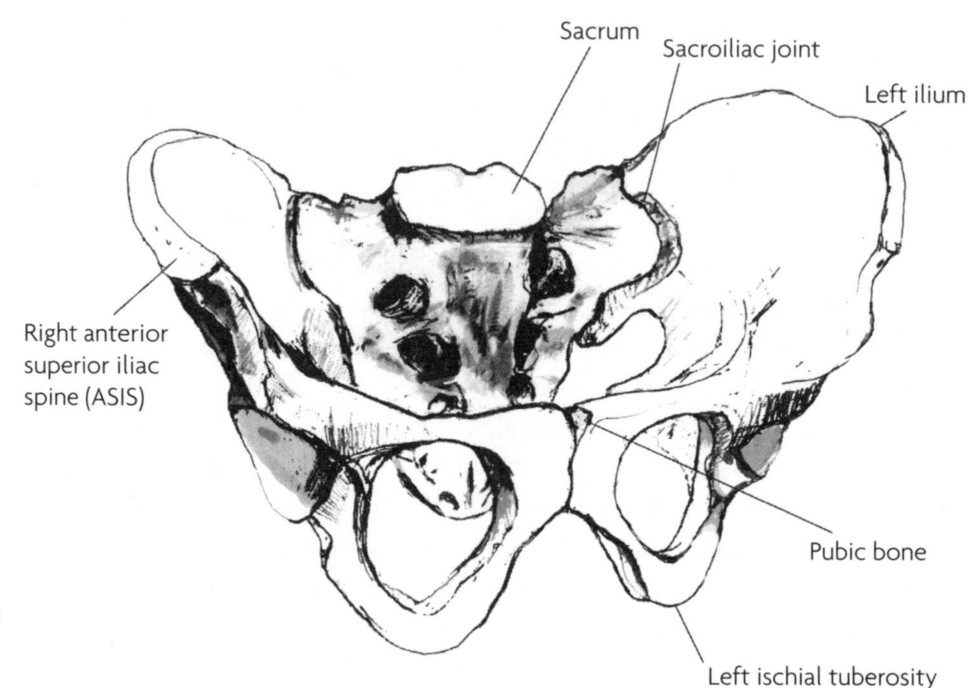

Fig. 2.2. A front view of the pelvis showing the relationship between the sacrum and the two ilia.

so that your eyes gaze straight upward. If your upper spine is rounded, lying flat may compress your throat when your head falls back. If this is true for you, place a folded towel under your neck and head. The support should allow your throat and airway to feel open. Have your hips and knees bent so that your feet are flat on the floor, legs parallel to one another and in line with your hip joints.

Press both feet evenly into the floor while reaching the tops of your shins forward, away from your hips. The movement is subtle and gradual. You will need only a few ounces of pressure through your feet. Your thighs should feel as though they are elongating away from your hips. Their motion will cause the top of your sacrum to roll back between the dimples, lifting your tailbone slightly away from the floor. To complete the movement, slowly relax your legs and allow your sacrum to settle back to your starting position. Imagine that your sacrum is soft enough to unfold from top to bottom.

If you have been taught an exercise called a pelvic lift, this practice may appear similar. However, there is an important distinction. In the pelvic lift, you use your buttocks and abdominal muscles to lift your hips from the floor. In the version described here, the pelvis does not lift up but rather rolls back. Keeping

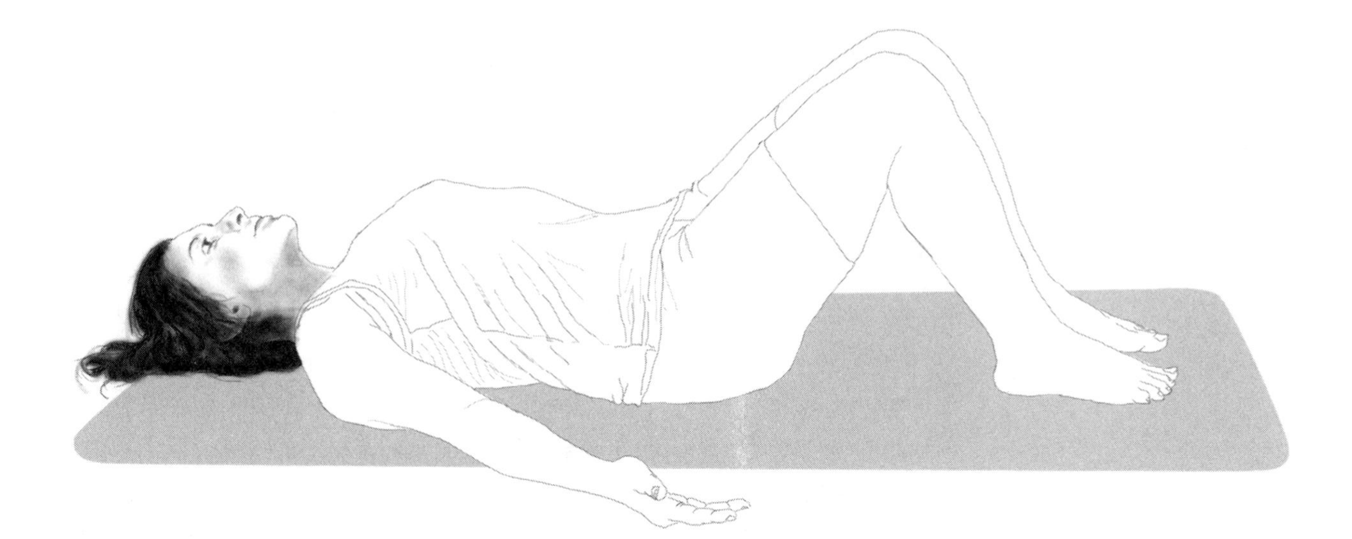

Fig. 2.3. Position for Sacroiliac Rocking practice.

the buttocks and abdominal muscles relaxed focuses the movement into the sacroiliac joints. Reaching forward through the upper shins is important. It stretches the muscles and fascia of the hips and pelvis so that your sacrum and ilia have room to articulate.

Rock your sacrum again. Press into your feet as you begin to exhale, completing the upward roll of the sacrum as you finish breathing out. Inhale with a soft belly and then, as you exhale again, gradually lower your sacrum to the starting position.

When you can feel your sacrum rocking, you're ready to alternate the motion from side to side. Press down into the floor with your right foot only and then reach forward through your right shin. As you do this, let your sacrum roll back into your left SI joint and dimple. Smoothly return to neutral and then reverse the movement. This time press down through your left foot, reach forward through your left shin, and roll back into your right SI joint. Again, return to neutral. Time your motions to coincide with slow, smooth exhalations.

You can picture the movement as a shallow "X" between each foot and its opposite SI joint. The movement should feel as though it is occurring inside your body and so subtly that someone across the room would not know you are moving. Your knees should travel forward no more than an inch as your sacrum rocks between the dimples. If you roll beyond the dimples onto the flesh of your buttocks you will not achieve the specific stretch of your sacroiliac joints. Instead, you'll be rocking your whole pelvis through your hip joints.

You may notice that it's easier to relax back into one sacroiliac joint than the other. Spend more time and attention on the restricted side. Imagine the tissues melting around the stiffer SI joint.

Exploration: Holistic Impact

To experience how tension travels through the connective tissue to distant regions of your body, try the following variant of the SI rocking exercise. Rock your sacrum as before while at the same time pursing your lips as if you are angry. Doing this will tighten muscles and fascia in your head, jaw, and throat.

Notice how much less motion is available in your lower spine and hips. Clenching your jaw may also have caused tension in your shoulders and arms. Every local muscle tension is communicated throughout the fascial internet. Even a small degree of that tension, adopted in daily life, will reduce the responsiveness of your whole body.

The more pliable your connective tissue, the more freely your muscles can move and the more adaptable your body will be to any movement you need to make, especially a sudden, unexpected one such as tripping over a child's toy left in the hall. If your body is articulate, you have a better chance of recovering your balance without injury. When any joint is restricted by thickened fascia, you can't move that part of your body freely. This reduces your ability to calibrate your balance. You are more likely to fall, and your tensed tissues are more likely to tear or break.

Slow-motion Exercise

When you practice Sacroiliac Rocking or any of several other slow-motion exercises in this book, you will encounter hesitations that keep your movement from being smooth. By going extremely slowly, you interrupt habitual tension around your sacroiliac joints. The hesitations indicate that your nervous system is revising the tension. If you rock quickly, you will not challenge your habit at the depth where change is needed.

Be sure to breathe steadily. Many people hold their breath when focusing intently. Release any tension that might have crept into your jaw, throat, hands, or feet. Be careful not to control the movement by pinching your buttocks together or by tucking your tailbone under. You will learn why this is important in chapter 3.

This meditative style of exercise is quite different from the "no pain, no gain" approach. Its purpose is to release habitual tensions rather than to increase strength or flexibility. Explore these exercises gently, never forcing and never pushing through any pain that you might encounter. Pain is a boundary to movement. By proceeding slowly and respectfully in relation to the boundary, you may gradually work through it. If you try to push through, you will make your tissues more defensive.

The rocking movement of your pelvis is also a massage for the organs that lie within your pelvic basin—your large and small intestines, reproductive organs, and bladder. These are all fluid, like sea creatures curled up within your lower abdomen. You may even hear a few gurgles within your belly as your movement redistributes pressures within your organs.

Time spent focusing on the sacrum can draw you into a state of heightened body awareness. In such a state, sensations in this region of your body may arouse deep emotions from early in life.

When we hold a newborn baby, our hands automatically cradle the tiny skull and sacrum with delicacy and awe. Our fingers touch the energetic foundations of the child's existence—the head and tail of the embryo from which new life has evolved. Sensitive contact at the sacrum, even for an adult, can evoke profound feelings of distress, if early life was threatened, or of peace, if early life experiences were secure. If moving your sacrum makes you feel weepy or vulnerable, do the practice in short sessions to build up tolerance for it. Restoring movement and sensation to this part of your body is integral to healing your posture.

Practice: Counterrotation of Pelvis and Chest

For this practice you simply continue Sacroiliac Rocking while focusing attention to your chest and upper spine. Notice that as you rock back into your left sacroiliac joint, your breastbone leans ever so slightly to the right. The breastbone and navel move in opposite directions. The displacement is very slight, a few degrees at most. You may prefer to sense the movement internally, noticing that as your intestines slide to the right, your heart rests slightly to the left.

Counterrotation of the upper and lower trunk is an important feature of healthy walking. If you find this difficult to feel, adopt Sacroiliac Rocking as a daily practice to prepare your spine for the healthy walking you will learn in chapter 9. The next practice, Curling and Arching, and others in ensuing chapters will also help free your spine.

Practice rocking your pelvis and letting your upper body rotate for several minutes. Then roll to one side and push yourself up to a sitting position. Get your bearings before you stand up. To complete the practice, walk around a bit, noticing sensations that are different from your "before" walk. These sensations may be specific to your sacrum or may occur at a distance from it. Some of you may feel shorter or closer to the ground. You may notice that your weight has become more evenly distributed over your feet. Your sacrum may feel more solid, more energized, or more vividly present. You may even feel a hint of rotation in your upper spine.

Practice: Curling and Arching

There are seventeen vertebrae in your spine, not including your neck. Each one should move independently of its neighbors. This practice evokes the forward and backward (*flexion* and *extension*) movements between vertebrae that are essential for healthy articulation of your spine. If possible, before you begin this exercise, ask a friend to massage the length of your spine, gently squeezing the vertebrae one by one. This will give you a fresh sensory experience of your spine.

Position yourself on hands and knees, palms directly below your armpits, knees directly below the creases of your groin. Spread your fingers so there is space between them and make firm contact between your hands and the floor. Feel the floor through the skin along your shins, ankles, and tops of your feet. (You'll discover the significance of skin surfaces in chapter 6.) If your ankles are too stiff to contact the floor, place a rolled towel under them. To keep from tucking your tailbone under, imagine your two sit bones spreading apart from one another. Relax your neck and allow your head to hang loosely downward.

Picture your vertebrae as seventeen jewels on an elastic necklace. You will be curling your spine toward the ceiling one jewel at a time. Begin with the jewel just below your neck and raise it toward the ceiling. As you do this, slightly increase the pressure of your palms into the floor. Raise each successive vertebra, counting slowly to seventeen. Keep firm skin contact on the floor with your fingers, palms,

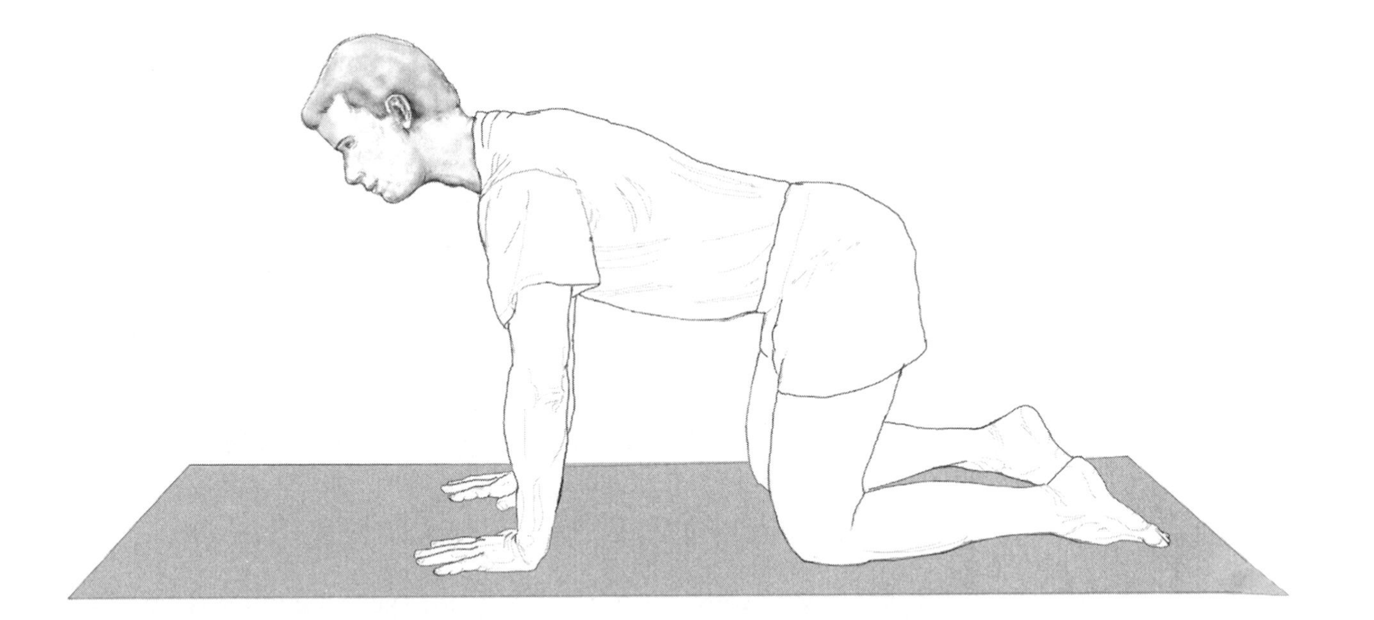

Fig. 2.4. Starting position for Curling and Arching practice.

shins, ankles, and toes. Imagine that the jewels are magnetized, each one individually attracted toward the ceiling. As you approach the lower vertebrae, your sacrum will curve downward. Maintain a sense of width between your sit bones to prevent the tendency to pinch your buttocks together. It may be difficult at first to feel the independent motion of each vertebra. Persist in visualizing them, giving each jewel a moment of attention.

Next, reverse the angle of your pelvis, allowing your tail to turn up. As this happens, the vertebra just above your sacrum will sink toward the floor. Lower your vertebrae one by one as if the jewels were now magnetized to the floor, counting slowly to seventeen as you proceed up your spine. Slowly raise your eyes toward the ceiling to reverse the curve in your neck. At the end, your spine will become a long downward arch from crown to tailbone.

Repeat the curling and arching, taking time to allow constricted muscles and connective tissue around your vertebrae to register the stretch. Breathe steadily throughout the movement and focus your breath into areas that feel tight. If you are aware that your spine is stiff, commit yourself to practicing this exercise for several minutes twice a day.

If you are uncomfortable kneeling, you can do this practice standing. Bend forward at the hips, relax your knees, and place your hands on a chair seat or tabletop.

Pedestrian Ballet

Our bodies are not machines. They are plastic, dynamic organisms, remnants of the sea encased on land. Healing posture involves restoring our bodies' ability to move freely yet efficiently—to move in ways that reconcile our need to move with our need for stability.

Let's look again at the pedestrians from this chapter's introduction. Elderly Mr. Carlsen's potbelly, arthritic joints, and halting gait all suggest a sedentary lifestyle, poor nutrition, and faulty breathing. Let's imagine him wandering into a senior center in the middle of a tai chi class. Let's imbue him with enough curiosity to cause him to stick around. The flowing, curvilinear movement of tai chi will send energy through his fascial pathways, invite him to breathe more efficiently, and do wonders for his mind as well as his body.

Bustling Mrs. Garcia is headed for a dowager's hump unless she joins the local YWCA and begins moving her shoulders and arms in ways that don't involve taking care of everyone else's problems. May she swim or belly dance her way to greater self-expression and healthier posture.

Rockie is currently blessed with flawless coordination, vitality, and grace. May he live and move in ways that preserve it. As for little Rico, we should hope that the school system fails to blunt his spirit enough to dull his delight in his body.

In part two, Stability, you will observe how tensions in the structures surrounding your internal organs can either support or distort your posture. You will begin, in chapter 3, by exploring the pelvic floor, which is the root of the interior channel along which stabilization occurs and the first of your healthy posture zones.

Part Two

Stability

The body is but a pair of pincers set over a bellows and a stewpan and the whole fixed upon stilts.

Samuel Butler,
nineteenth-century British author

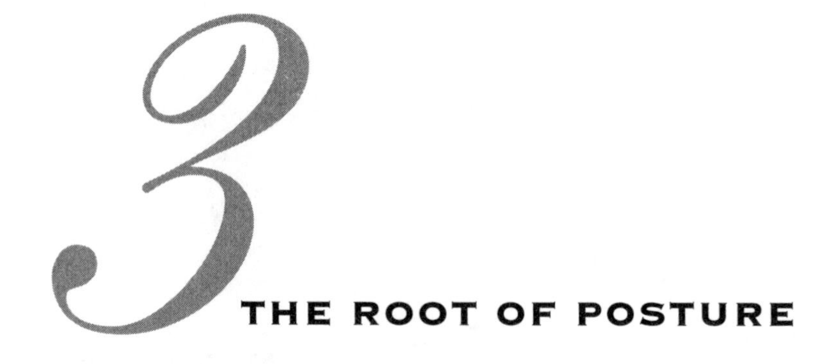

3 THE ROOT OF POSTURE

In this chapter, you will explore the first of your six posture zones, the "floor" of your pelvis. Sitting down is the easiest position in which to become aware of this region of your body, so the chapter also addresses healthy sitting. By learning the secret of sitting, you reconcile your body's design for movement with the reality of a sedentary workplace. Balance in the pelvic floor also affects the mobility of your spine and legs and is therefore essential for healthy walking. Further, the pelvic floor is the root of abdominal support and healthy breathing.

Our own physical body possesses a wisdom which we who inhabit the body lack. We give it orders which make no sense.

Henry Miller

Alison's Ergonomic Chair

Last month, after getting news of her promotion, Alison splurged on an expensive ergonomic chair. In the past year, she'd spent a fortune on medical tests, physical therapy, and painkilling drugs. In the long run, she figured, the chair would save money.

The pain was a mystery. Alison hadn't been in any car accidents, had never even broken a bone. She kept in shape with yoga and running. Lately, though, she had been going to the office on weekends. The pain in her back was always worse after that.

Alison is a willowy blonde. She put herself through design school doing runway modeling and still walks like a model, with her hips thrust forward. Her chest caves in a little, but she's so pretty that people don't find it unattractive.

It's been six weeks now and she's frustrated. She's tried every one of the chair's adjustable features—seat angle, armrest height, lumbar support, and headrest position. Initially each new setting feels comfy. Ahh, that's it. But within an hour her body is aching, a prisoner of the chair.

The amazing achievements of the technological age—from laser surgery to video phones—seduce us into thinking that every problem can be solved by a gadget. Alison's chair supports her body in what seems like good alignment. However, with all its bells and whistles, the chair cannot address the root of her problem—the tension around her pelvic floor.

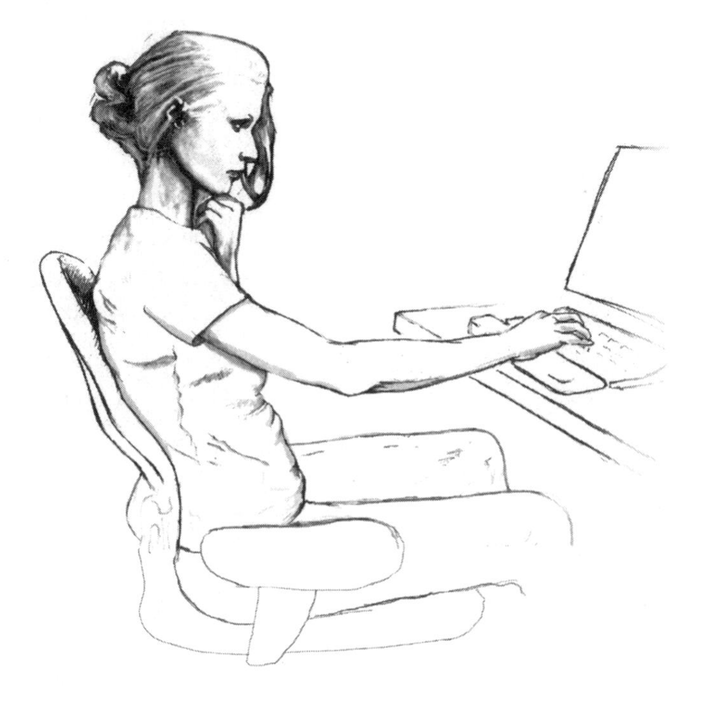

Fig. 3.1. Alison's chair positions her chest behind her pelvis, putting strain on her lower back, chest, shoulders, and neck.

Alison's tucked-under pelvis has less to do with modeling than with landing hard on her tailbone when she was twelve years old. Her brother pushed her out of a tree. Rather than complain, she suffered in silence because she wasn't supposed to be out playing. The incident left a residue of pelvic tension that is charged with childhood shame and anger. Because of this seemingly minor incident, Alison has protected this area of her body for twenty years. She sits too far back on her pelvis, so the most elaborate ergonomics design on earth cannot support her. Her habitual tension sabotages her body's orientation.

Alison is not alone in suffering from the way she sits. Seventy percent of Americans spend most of their waking lives sitting behind a steering wheel or in front of a computer screen. Whether their work is a joy or a chore, most of them are uncomfortable.

Prolonged sitting is associated with a long list of physical complaints. The C-curved, slouching posture of most sedentary workers puts uneven pressure on spinal discs, irritating nerves and sparking back pain. Because such posture compresses the internal organs, it can also be related to digestive and urogenital problems. In addition, because the diaphragm cannot fully descend when the abdomen is compressed, the upper chest breathing that results can lead to problems created by breathing dysfunction.

Slouching causes the head to jut forward and strains the joints between the neck and upper back. This can result in an unattractive buildup of fascia which collects to stabilize the misaligned vertebrae. The forward head position also compresses the joints between the neck and head, causing tension headaches and poor concentration. Further, a forward head posture compresses the area between the collarbone and arms, restricting nerves and blood vessels that supply the hands and leading to hand and wrist pain, weakness, numbness, or tingling.

Ergonomics researchers agree that sedentary workers' complaints are directly related to sitting posture. Every year sees new chair designs based on revised assessments of seat contour and inclination, the angle of the seat back, chair height, and adjustability. While chair designers have studied the body, they are missing two important facts about human structure. First, the body is not engineered to sit still but to be in motion. Second, the posture that leads to most complaints begins with inadequate support from the pelvis.

Alison's chair has a double-contoured seat meant to separately cradle each thigh and buttock. The contouring prevents her from making the squirming movements that keep the tension in her spine at bay. However, she'd been taught since age six that sitting still was proper, so it was easy to be talked into buying a chair that actually gave her too much support.

Alison needs to sit in a way that removes pressure from her tailbone, frees her spine and rib cage for breathing, and allows efficient bending and reaching as she performs her tasks. Her comfort and support depend not solely on chair design but also on changes she must make in the orientation of her pelvis.

Understanding Your Pelvis

To see why your pelvic floor is so crucial to healthy posture, you need to understand the relationship between your pelvis and spine. The pelvis is a two-tiered basin. The sacrum, which you explored in chapter 2, is its back wall. If you are not familiar with human anatomy, the three-dimensional contours of the pelvis can be difficult to visualize. The best way to grasp the shape of the pelvis is to get your hands on one. The following paragraphs walk you through a simple self-palpation.

EXPLORATION: PELVIS PALPATION

As you did in chapter 2, place your third fingers on the dimples near your sacroiliac joints. Then extend the webbing between your thumbs and index fingers along the bony crests just below your waist. Slide your thumbs forward along these crests until each thumb comes to a promontory.

This point is commonly but inaccurately known as the hip bone. Its anatomical name is *anterior superior iliac spine* or, for short, *ASIS.* With your thumb at this promontory and the webbing and heels of your hands resting along the crests, let your fingers slide down to cover the broad, wing-shaped ilia that form the side walls of your lower belly.

Now slip your thumbs forward over the two ASISs and down into the creases between your pelvis and legs. Here the ilia connect to two branches of bone that merge in the center of your pelvis to form your *pubic bone.* From back to front, the sacrum, two ilia, and pubic bone form the rim of a shallow upper basin into which the fascial bag that contains your intestines rests.

The lower tier of the pelvic basin is formed by two crescent-shaped bones that project down from beneath the sacroiliac joints and merge with the underside of the pubic bone. Place your right hand between your legs and reach back to touch your left sit bone. Then walk your fingertips forward along a bony rim to your groin. Feel how the rim merges with your pubic bone.

This part of the pelvis is called the *ischium.* The two rims border the lower tier of the pelvis, a small basin about the size of a large cappuccino mug. The two

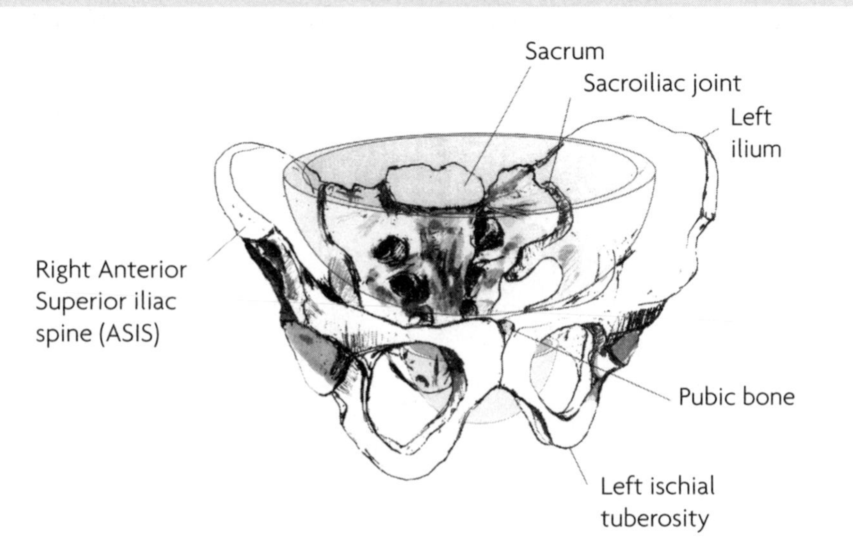

Fig. 3.2. A female pelvis, showing the upper and lower pelvic basins. Male pelvises are taller and narrower.

knobs at the bottom of the rims, the *ischial tuberosities,* are the sit bones. Your bladder rests in the lower pelvic basin. In women, the uterus lies just above the bladder. In men, the seminal vesicles and prostate nestle behind and below it. The angle at which the pelvis sits on the tuberosities can affect the function of these pelvic organs.

Roll your pelvis backward across your sit bones toward your tailbone, then forward over the ischial rims toward your pubic bone. This rolling motion takes place through your hip joints. Your thighbones, or *femurs,* have rounded tops about the size of a Ping-Pong ball (the "head" of the femur) which fit into recessed sockets near the bottom of each wing of your ilia. When you rock your pelvis back and forth, you are rotating your ilia around the femoral heads.

YOUR PELVIC DIAMOND

The pelvic floor, sometimes called the *perineum,* is a diamond-shaped area defined by four bony landmarks—the two sit bones, the pubic bone, and the coccyx (tailbone). A muscular sling extends across the area and divides it into two triangles. The one in front is called the *urogenital triangle;* the one in back is the *anal triangle*. Because it is penetrated by the urethra, vagina, and anus, the pelvic floor is the outlet for the visceral core of the body.

The pelvic floor muscles draw inward and upward to prevent urinary flow. Most women have learned to duplicate this action as an exercise called the Kegel. Named after obstetrician Arnold Kegel, the movement helps restore function when pelvic floor tissues have been damaged in childbirth. Many people—and not just women—have solved either sexual dysfunction

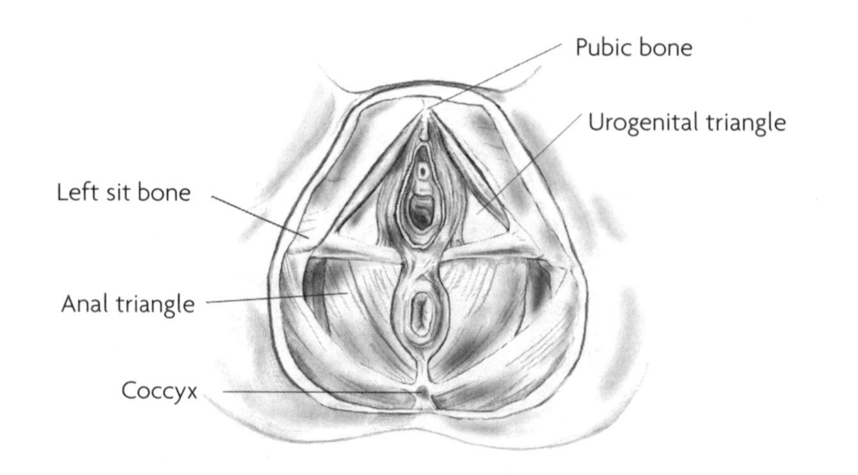

Fig. 3.3. The diamond-shaped female pelvic floor, showing the front and back triangles. Male pelvic floors also have this shape.

or urinary incontinence by strengthening the perineal muscles. In chapter 5 you will explore Kegel's exercise in conjunction with support for your abdomen.

It is important to distinguish between the muscles of the pelvic floor and those immediately surrounding it. Activity in the perineum itself does not change the inclination of the pelvis, but because the bones defining the pelvic floor are attached to muscles of the buttocks and thighs, tension in these muscles does affect the orientation of the pelvic floor. The following explorations will help you experience different orientations of your pelvis when you are sitting.

Exploration: The Pelvic Floor Diamond

Sit on an office or a dining room chair without leaning against the chair back. Then contract your buttocks and the backs of your thighs. Notice how this action rolls your whole pelvis backward. Your weight now rests through the back triangle, tailbone, and lower buttocks. Your sit bones seem to have moved closer together, narrowing the anal triangle.

Now relax the contraction of your buttocks and thighs and roll your pelvis forward so that your trunk is poised over the front triangle. This seems to spread your sit bones slightly apart from each other and tips your pubic bone down toward the seat. Your weight now rests on the back of your upper thighs, just in front of your sit bones. Notice also that the tiny space between your anus and coccyx has lengthened. There is a tiny ligament here, the *anococcygeal ligament.*

Exploration: The Anal Triangle

For many people, relaxation of the anococcygeal area is the single most important key to healing their posture. The movements of this exploration are so slight that someone watching you might not notice that you are moving, but the difference in the tension of your pelvic floor can have far-reaching effects on your spine and overall posture.

Shorten the space between your anus and coccyx by imagining your anococcygeal ligament getting very short. Notice how this makes your pelvis roll slightly backward. Now reverse the direction. Imagine that space lengthening to allow

Sitting on a Ball

Sitting on a large exercise ball is a great way to enhance awareness of your pelvic floor and relax your pelvis and hips. Have the ball less than fully inflated so that it presents a cushy, feel-good surface. Pretend the ball is an old-fashioned inkpad and that your buttocks and thighs are a rubber stamp. Imbue every inch of the stamp with ink by rolling your pelvis around on the ball. Do this slowly so that the movement of your pelvis, spine, and hips feels smooth, curving, and continuous. Plant your feet firmly on the floor so there is no danger of the ball rolling out from under you.

This practice involves entrusting your weight to the ball. To adapt to the unstable yet inviting surface, you must release any tensions in your hips, legs, and pelvis. Once you feel comfortable letting the ball support you, try to find similar sensations of support when sitting in an ordinary chair.

more room in the anal triangle. This lets your pelvis roll forward so that your pubic bone can rest down.

Repeat the exploration. This time, pay attention to corresponding changes in the curve of your lower back. When you roll back, closing the anal triangle, your lower back flattens, your chest drops, and your feet probably feel more lightly placed on the floor. However, when your pelvic floor is open, your lower back curves forward, your chest lifts, and your legs and feet will likely feel grounded. Notice also that this open orientation of your pelvic floor can make it easier to breathe. This short exploration demonstrates how one posture zone affects the others.

Shouldn't My Spine Be Straight?

By now, you will have noticed that the curve of the lower back changes with different inclinations of the pelvis. Healthy sitting calls for a slight forward tilt of the pelvis. This inclination causes a gentle forward curve of the lower back, which many of us have been taught is wrong. To understand the structural logic of the forward pelvic alignment, we need to correct some misconceptions about the mechanics of our spines.

When a standing body is well aligned, gravity's vector travels through its central core. Most of you have seen illustrations of good posture in which the ear, tip of a shoulder, and centers of the hip, knee, and ankle joints are plumb. For many years, physical educators taught vertical alignment by positioning the spine itself in a straight line. Students were taught to flatten their backs against a wall. While well-educated fitness professionals no longer use this approach, it still influences cultural beliefs about posture.

The twenty-four vertebrae of the spine overlap one another like shingles. Their individual contours and articulations give the spine three natural curves. The shape of the two forward curves—with the convex surfaces facing front—is called *lordosis*. They occur in the *cervical vertebrae* of the neck and the *lumbar vertebrae* of the lower back. The concavity of the upper back is called *kyphosis*.

The curves in the spine provide shock absorption. If you walk with a pronounced heel strike, every step sends an impact up and into the spine. By distributing the pressures of locomotion, the curvatures help prevent damage to the vertebral discs (the cartilaginous cushions between vertebrae) and protect the delicate internal organs that are suspended from the front of the spine.

Some of you may have heard the words *kyphosis* and *lordosis* used to describe poor posture. Kyphosis or lordosis become problems when extreme curvatures are so set by habitual muscular tension and accompanying fascial adhesion that the spine loses resilience and adaptability. People may become unable to straighten kyphotic areas or to bend lordotic areas. The curves themselves are beneficial. They are dysfunctional only when they become extreme or too stiff to move.

Restriction in any one of the curvatures creates compensatory tension in muscles and fascia of the curves above or below. Also, because the sacrum—the base of the spine—is the back of the pelvis, the inclination of the pelvis also affects the curvatures.

When you rock your pelvis back toward your anal triangle, diminishing your natural lordosis, this position of your pelvis is called backward tilt.

Fig. 3.4. Pelvic tilt in standing postures (left to right: backward tilt, forward tilt, and a neutral position). Notice how pelvic tilt affects the curve of the lumbar spine.

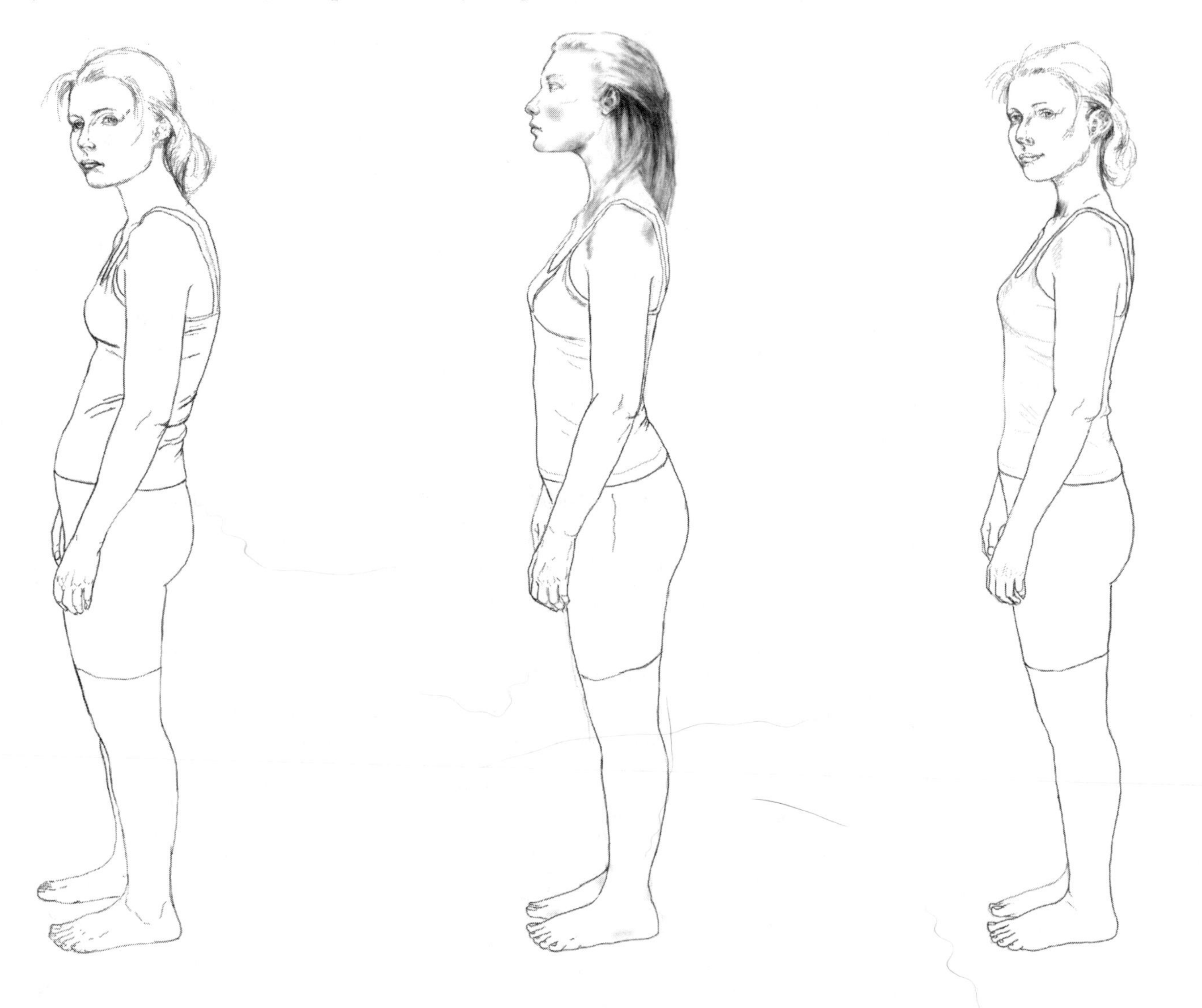

Sitting or standing with a backward pelvic tilt for extended periods of time puts uneven pressure on the lumbar disks, unduly stretches the sacroiliac joints, stresses spinal muscles, and compromises the curves in the upper spine and neck. This is the inevitable result of stabilizing the trunk by closing the pelvic floor.

When you rock your pelvis forward toward the urogenital triangle, you increase your lumbar lordosis. This angle of the pelvis is known as forward pelvic tilt. Exaggerated forward tilt compresses the lumbar vertebrae and prevents them from articulating properly, but a mild forward tilt gives the lumbar vertebrae the best mechanical advantage for both stability and movement. A gentle curve is the neutral position for the lumbar spine.

Healthy Sitting

Because chairs are ubiquitous in Western culture, we assume that sitting in them is natural. Ancient humans, however, did not sit in chairs. Their lives were a constant flow of physical activity—walking, hunting, gathering food, and setting up and breaking down camps. For domestic tasks, they knelt or squatted, and when they were tired they lay down. They had no chairs and, most likely, no back pain.

In studies of present-day societies in which people squat rather than sit on chairs, researchers have found lower rates of spinal disc degeneration than in societies in which people sit in chairs.* In modern America, no one older than the age of four squats. Our hips aren't flexible enough to squat because we spend too much time in chairs and too little time using our bodies the way they were designed to be used.

Because your body is engineered for movement, you can't expect to sit through fifty-hour weeks without suffering some consequences. However, three factors can help you do it with minimum damage to your body:

- Awareness of the best use of your anatomy while you sit.
- A chair that fits your body and fosters good body use.
- The better your basic health and fitness, the more adaptable your body will be to the abuse of prolonged sitting. If your work requires prolonged sitting, you have as much need to stay in shape as an athlete.

We'll discuss the first two factors in this chapter. We look at exercise in chapter 10.

*Galen Cranz, *The Chair: Rethinking Culture, Body, and Design* (New York: W. W. Norton & Company, 1998), 98.

Exploration: Slouching

Find a chair with a firm, flat surface, neither contoured nor thickly padded. It should be tall enough that your hips are higher than your knees when you are sitting. Place a telephone book or folded towel in the seat pan if it is contoured or if the chair is too low. Put the phone book under your feet if the chair is too high. Sit on the chair as if it were a bench; don't lean against the backrest.

To begin, take a discriminating tour of the typical C-curved slouch. Go ahead and slouch as you might at the end of a long day. Notice that your body's weight falls to the back edge of your sit bones. Your coccyx tucks under, narrowing the space between your sit bones and closing your pelvic floor. Your lumbar lordosis flattens, and you may feel strain in your sacroiliac joints. Your feet have very light contact with the floor because your legs are not contributing to your base of support. Your foundation consists of the small area between your sit bones and sacrum.

Your shoulders will have rounded and your sternum dropped so that your rib cage seems to be resting on your abdomen. This leaves little room for your intestines, which now press outward against your abdominal wall. Notice also that your head leans forward in front of your chest and that this creates a bulge at the rear base of your neck. When you turn your head to look behind you from this position, you aren't able to see very far.

Notice that you can't take a full, easy breath. Your diaphragm is prevented from descending by the abdomen below, and your ribs can't rise because of pressure from the neck and shoulders above.

Many people assume that a slouched sitting posture is due to laziness and that the old admonitions—"sit up straight" and "shoulders back"—are all they need to put it right. However, as long as your pelvis is tilted back, you won't be comfortable with an erect trunk for more than a few minutes. Unless your base of support can be transferred forward, nothing you do to improve the configuration of your upper body will be sustainable. Although it's true that underactive spinal muscles contribute to poor posture, the main cause of poor sitting posture is lack of support from the pelvis and legs. The key to finding this support is the sensation of spaciousness in your pelvic diamond.

Pelvic Health

Because good seated posture balances tensions in the pelvic region, healthy sitting contributes to your overall health. An unconscious instinct to protect the genitals and rectum causes many of us to carry tension within the perineum or in surrounding buttocks muscles. Almost everyone has experienced some degree of trauma to this vulnerable area, be it an event so mundane as falling off a bicycle or something as traumatic as sexual abuse. Our bodies need protection here. But constant tension around the pelvic floor can result in chronic pelvic pain, urinary urgency, rectal pain, and sexual dysfunction. In many cases, these symptoms are relieved by reducing pelvic floor tension.*

*David Wise, Ph.D., and Rodney U. Anderson, M.D., *A Headache in the Pelvis* (Occidental, Calif.: National Center for Pelvic Pain Research, 2003), 81.

Exploration: Supported Sitting

To come out of the slouch, simply roll your pelvis forward so that you feel your anal triangle widening and your pubic bone dropping. Stop when your pubic bone and coccyx are on the same horizontal plane. The change in your foundation will distribute your weight slightly in front of your sit bones, with part of your weight on your thighs. About 60 percent of your weight will be distributed through your pelvis and 40 percent through your legs and feet. This 60/40 balance means that your base of support is deep, spanning the entire area between your heels and sit bones.

Allow your spine, chest, and shoulders to adjust to the change in your foundation. Your lumbar spine should now curve forward, generating a lift in your chest and throat. This in turn supports a more elevated positioning of your head. Notice that you can see farther behind you when you turn your neck from this position.

With your weight resting on your legs, there is no pressure on your sacrum or coccyx. Instead, your sacrum rests between the ilia in a way that stabilizes the sacroiliac joints. The slight lumbar curve gives your abdominal organs more space in which to function. With your diaphragm now free to descend, you also have more breathing room.

Sitting with a slight lumbar lordosis gives your body its broadest base of support. When you are seated forward, your legs feel weighted and your feet seem to have better connection with the ground.

Healthy sitting requires that your body be adaptable in the hips, spine, chest, shoulders, and neck. If you have tight muscles in the backs of your legs, you may find that tilting the pelvis forward strains your hips or lower back. You may also be aware that because your chest cannot rise, the pelvis has no room to roll forward. If healthy sitting isn't comfortable right away, practice it to whatever extent you can. Little by little, your muscles and fascia will accommodate to your new orientation, especially as you restore balance to the other healthy posture zones. Continued discomfort means that your body needs exercise, bodywork, or both.

Your Diamond in Daily Life

From picking up a child's toy to teeing up a golf ball and from brushing your teeth to hefting a grocery bag, bending over and straightening up are actions you make countless times a day. Correct performance of these simple actions is essential to the health of your spine. Knowing how to bend and straighten correctly from a seated position can help you understand how to do these actions right when you're standing.

Most people reach for things by bending over from the waist, with their chest and shoulders folding inward. Bending over in this manner is the inevitable result of sitting too far back in the pelvic diamond. Straightening up from this position strains muscles in the lower back. If, instead, you begin your action from the 60/40 balance we have been developing, you will find that you can lean your torso forward by using your hip joints as hinges. When you tip forward this way, you will feel your body weight transferred down your legs into your feet. Then, when you straighten up, you can use your legs for leverage.

Exploration: Bending Over

Sit so that your pelvic floor diamond is open, with the back triangle released. Have your knees in line with your hips. Place your feet on the floor so that your ankles are just in front of your knees. Take a few easy breaths, widening your lower rib cage and letting your breath fill both the front and back of your lungs. Then lean your torso forward by letting your hip joints fold like hinges. Allow the space between your sit bones to widen as you move forward. Feel your coccyx rising up, away from the chair, and your pubic bone tilting down.

Notice that you can lean forward without having to round your back or compress your abdomen. If this action feels awkward, check whether you might have unconsciously braced your buttocks muscles and closed your pelvic floor. Relax, letting your weight settle into the chair, and try the forward lean again.

To return to an upright position, lightly push your feet down into the floor. At the same time, imagine that you are gently pressing the floor forward, away from you. This action reopens the creases of your hips and stimulates the extensor muscles of your spine. Notice how holistic the action is. Instead of overstressing your lower back muscles, you use your legs and spine to regain the upright position.

If you have experienced injury to your pelvic floor or tailbone, bending over in this manner can make you feel vulnerable. It may take you some time to get used to the feeling of relaxing the closure around your anal triangle.

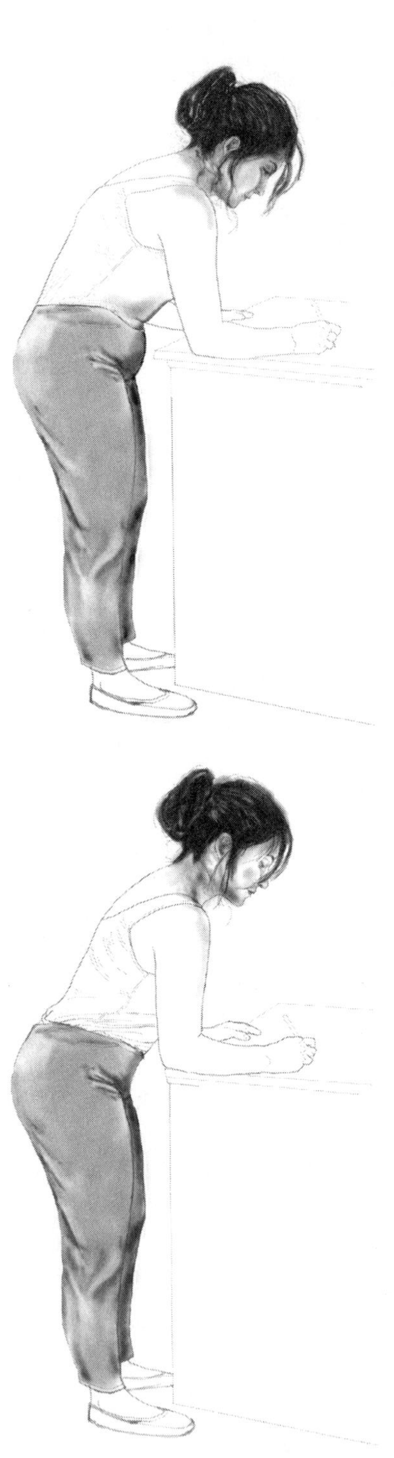

Fig. 3.5. By releasing her pelvic floor and hips, Carmen has changed the way she bends over.

Experiment with a simple task that involves writing. Use your sacrum and hip joints to incline your body toward your writing surface. You do not have to curl yourself into a ball whenever you sign your name.

Try bending over from a standing position. The tendency to tighten the posterior triangle is usually more pronounced when you bend over while standing. Choose several daily activities that involve bending over and revise them to incorporate your new awareness of space around your tailbone. Experiment while you put on your pants, make the bed, or pick up children's toys.

In later chapters, we will explore the role of the pelvic floor in standing and walking. If it is already easy for you to sustain a sense of the open diamond as you walk, go ahead and practice this. If the new breadth in your derriere makes walking feel awkward, this is because there are fascial and muscular restrictions in your hips and spine that have yet to be addressed. As healthy sitting becomes more comfortable, the open diamond will gradually feel more natural in walking as well.

For Carmen, the cashier from Target with a backache, awareness of the pelvic floor diamond was an initiation into a whole new consciousness about her body. She realized she'd always felt embarrassed about her derriere. Whenever she cheated on her diet, the pounds all went right there. She'd developed the habit of tensing her buttocks to make herself feel thinner. Now she could sense how this habit blocked her hip joints, which, in turn strained her back when she did much bending over. Relaxing the tension around her coccyx felt odd at first, as if she were putting herself on display, but if changing that little habit could stop the pain, she'd give it a try.

Exploration: Perceptual Fine Tuning

In chapter 1, we began to explore the relationship between sensory perceptions and posture. Recall that when you thought about a simple pleasure, your posture became more open. The link between perception and posture also works the other way around: If your body is well supported, that affects your outlook on the world around you. Take a few minutes to observe differences in your perceptions while seated in various postures.

Begin by sitting in your habitual way. Imagine yourself in a social context—a business lunch, perhaps. Notice your attitude toward others when you sit in a slouched posture. Then change your base of support by reorienting your pelvis, legs, and spine. Notice how your body position changes your perception of the situation. Possible variations in your viewpoint might include curiosity, interest, and openness rather than boredom, guardedness, or judgment. Of course, the true test will come when you experiment in real time with real people.

Now imagine a hostile situation. In which seated posture do you feel more grounded and resourceful?

By practicing healthy sitting, you support the opening of your perceptions. Also, by adopting the sensations and viewpoints that correlate with healthy sitting, you develop your perceptual template for sitting well. This helps you revamp your coordination and strengthen your muscles so that, in time, sitting poorly will become physically uncomfortable. It will also become emotionally uncomfortable.

Chairs and Compromises

Eighty-five percent of us will experience back pain sometime in our lives. Complaints about back pain have soared as our workplaces have become more sedentary. It is certain that these two trends are related. If we remember that our bodies are designed for movement, it should come as no surprise that prolonged sitting is harmful to our health. Learning to use your anatomy to your best advantage helps prevent problems caused by sedentary occupations. Your body's growing demand for the sensations of healthy support will help you select a chair that provides it. Having the right chair can make a huge difference in your day.

Ergonomics researchers base their analysis of good seating on what happens to the body when it is floating in zero gravity or in water. When the body is floating, there is a wide angle between the trunk and thighs, approximately 135 degrees. Research suggests that this position—basically how you sit in a lounge chair—puts the least possible pressure on lumbar disks. It also involves minimal energy expenditure by the back muscles.

Designs for modern office chairs incorporate this wide hip angle by inclining seat backs away from seats. The resulting semireclined position makes a person thrust his neck forward in order to keep the head upright. This puts undue tension on neck muscles. Designers solve this problem by making the upper part of the seat concave. Although this C-curve in the seat back lets the neck be supported by the upper trunk, it also pushes the chest

Car Seats

Car seat designers attempt to accommodate the average body. Because few people sit with good pelvic support, car seats are molded around the average person's poor posture. This means that achieving good support in your car requires some ingenuity.

Adjust your seat back to be as upright as possible. To sit with a spacious pelvic floor, slide your buttocks as far back as you can into the crack between the backrest and seat. The bottom of the seat back can then support your sacrum. This arrangement will leave several inches of space between your spine and the seat back. Insert a cushion or other prop into this space to support your chest. A prop in the lumbar area may be comfortable for some people, although placing it higher up, just below the shoulder blades, will feel better for others. A small bolster filled with buckwheat hulls can be moved up or down to accommodate your spine's shifting tensions on long drives.*

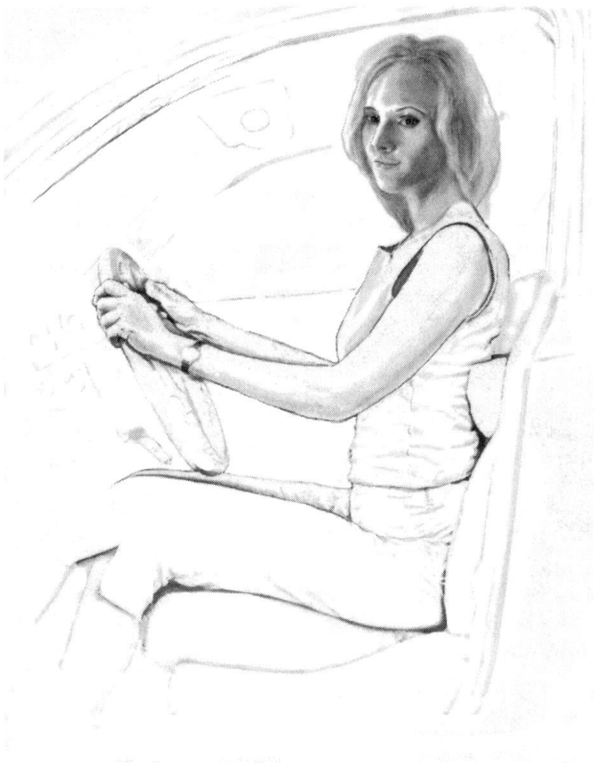

When the prop is positioned correctly, your torso should feel taller and more open and your neck should be comfortably centered above your heart. You may find that this thrusts the top of your head nearer to the car's roof. The next time you buy a car, be sure it fits your best posture. The greater height of SUVs, vans, and trucks offers sufficient headroom to allow for sitting with your spine and chest erect. The height also allows for a more open groin angle. Seats in small cars incline back, compressing the body to fit inside and forcing the chest back and neck forward.

Make time to interrupt prolonged sitting, in car or office, with periods of physical activity. For long road trips, add five minutes per hour to your estimated arrival time and stop long enough to work the kinks out of your body.

*See the appendix for suggestions about using props for sitting.

Fig. 3.6. By finding spaciousness through her pelvic floor and placing a small bolster just below her shoulder blades, Alison finds a comfortable way to sit in her car.

down onto the abdomen, compressing the internal organs and restricting breathing. The C-curve also flattens the lumbar spine, a problem solved by adding a forward curve to the lumbar area of the seat back. This lumbar support further displaces the chest behind the base of support. This vicious circle of design flaws rests on a basic ergonomic fallacy—that the problem of sitting can be solved by chair design alone.

You will have noticed that the section on healthy sitting made no mention of a backrest. A healthy spine is perfectly engineered to support the trunk. If the spine requires no backrest in the standing position, why should it require support when you are seated? The spine has no need to lean back on anything as long as the pelvis and legs provide a broad enough base of support.

Belief that the spine needs support is based on an assumption that the body must be protected from gravity, a misunderstanding of the body's engineering. Our bodies are designed to interact dynamically with gravity through our movements. Muscular activity helps dissipate the toxic biochemical effects of stress. In addition, the effects of gravity keep our bones and muscles healthy. Astronauts risk osteoporosis and muscular atrophy after just three months in zero gravity.

Backrests come into play because our twenty-first-century bodies have spent lifetimes sitting in chairs. For most people, adapting to sitting without back support will take time. During the interim, you need optional back support. Most ergonomic office chairs provide lumbar support. However, padding meant to support your spine's natural curve can cause the reverse effect. The sensation of the lumbar cushion may make you press your spine into the support and decrease your lumbar curve.

The best way to protect your lower back while sitting is to have support above and below the lumbar area. If you have a standard office chair, adjust the seat back or lumbar cushion downward until it provides light pressure on your sacrum. This will support your pelvis, which is the root of seated posture. When the sacrum feels supported, the spine above it responds with an automatic lift. Lumbar support only addresses the spine, not the pelvis. Some of you may appreciate additional support just below the shoulder blades, to elevate the chest and support the diaphragm.

Consider the following factors when selecting or adapting a chair for your workplace:

- The chair seat should be adjustable to a height that allows your hip joints to be slightly higher than your knees. This means that your thighs

But My Belly Sticks Out!

You may find that sitting with a neutral lordotic curve and bending over with a spacious pelvic floor makes you aware of a protruding abdomen, especially if you carry excess weight there. The fault is not the new sitting posture or new way of bending over but that you lack tone in the muscles that contain and stabilize your core. This was Carmen's problem in the introduction. You'll find her solution and yours in chapter 5.

will be inclined downward and your hip angle will be greater than 90 degrees.

- Fill in overly cushioned or contoured seats with firm material.
- To maintain your lumbar curve, try a seat wedge. This is a foam pad with the back 20 percent higher than the front, available at ergonomics retailers.
- Select a chair that has enough space between the seat and back for your buttocks to swell into. In chairs with a flush angle between the back and seat, the buttocks are pressed forward by the seat back and the pelvis gradually slides forward on the seat. This tilts the pelvis back and puts your weight onto your sacrum. Some seats prevent sliding with a raised front edge, but this tactic only increases posterior pelvic tilt by raising the thighs.
- Adjust the seat back to support your pelvis rather than your lumbar spine.
- If you decide to buy an ergonomic chair, be sure there's a generous return policy. You won't know how well the chair fits you until you sit and work in it for a while.*

Adjust your work surfaces to accommodate your new sitting height. Your forearms should incline slightly from your elbows, wrists in line with your forearms as your fingers touch the keyboard. Avoid using armrests. In healthy sitting, the shoulders are supported by your spine, eliminating the need for arm or wrist support. Leaning on armrests encourages the shoulders to roll forward, which closes the chest and compresses the spine. Use armrests only for periods of "R & R." Your eyes should be level with the top third of your computer screen. If this puts you so high that your feet dangle, you'll need a footrest to ground your feet.

Exploration: Smart Reclining

For moments at work when you kick back for socializing or introspection, it's fine to rest into the back of your chair, but learn to do it without compromising your pelvic floor. The trick is to lean on the backrest without rolling your pelvis back and flattening your lumbar curve. You can do this by leaning straight back from your hips. The action is the reverse of what you did to bend forward into activity. In this case you are leaning away from activity.

*See the appendix for a list of chairs that support healthy sitting.

Try it now. Start from the healthy sitting position with your buttocks well back into the seat angle but not leaning on the backrest at first. Then lean your upper torso straight back. When your upper back contacts the backrest, let your lumbar area relax. This approach preserves a slight degree of lumbar lordosis. You'll know you've done it correctly if you feel your weight being born through your sit bones when you lean back, not through your sacrum or coccyx. The pelvic diamond remains spacious. The posture should feel open through your abdomen and diaphragm.

Body Fashion

You may find that other people will regard your new erect posture as an affectation. "Gee, you sure have great posture," can be said in a derogatory tone, as if to make you wrong for choosing how to occupy your body. Because we all want connection with others, we may be swayed from our personal perception of what feels right. There are fashions in body postures just as there are fashions in clothing, cars, or chair designs. Current body fashion espouses a cool and casual yet intense look. Slouching is "in."

As you heal your posture, your body will gradually become taller, more open, more centered, and more powerful. Your new look may even be intimidating to some people. Let the choice of how to organize your body be dictated by your own perceptions rather than by someone else's judgment.

In frustration, Alison did a Google search for "correct sitting" and found a helpful article at www.newrulesofposture.com. When she read the part about a diamond at the root of her pelvis, a light bulb went on. For years she'd heard yoga instructors say, "Spread the sit bones," but now she realized the instruction wasn't just for yoga practice but also for life in general. The tiny adjustment of that little ligament "down there" let her feel both stable and open. The posture reminded her of sitting astride a horse. She had a feeling of command combined with a sense of easy mobility. She sat that way on her old office chair for the next week without taking a single painkiller.

The only problem now was that her new ergonomic chair didn't fit her new posture. Fortunately there was a sixty-day return policy on the chair. Alison let out a sigh of relief. The new orientation of her pelvic floor even made it easier to breathe. She had always suspected she didn't "breathe right." Alison is not alone in wondering about her breathing. Chapter 4 explores your next key to healthy posture—healthy breathing.

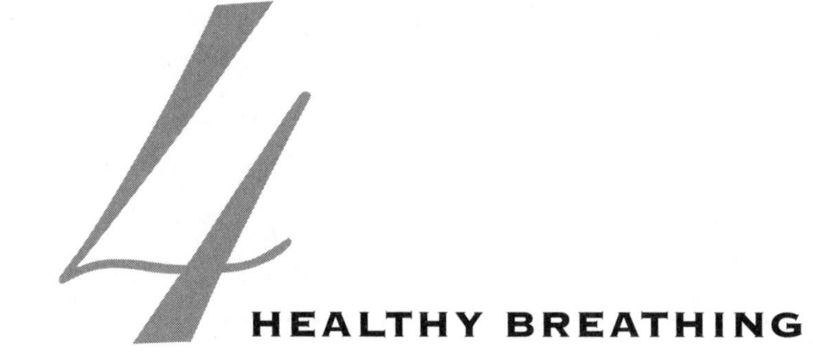

HEALTHY BREATHING

And the Lord God formed man of the dust of the ground, and breathed into his nostrils the breath of life; and man became a living soul.

GENESIS 2:7

You must fall in love with your own breath. Then you can begin to learn to love others.

ADNAN SARHAN, CONTEMPORARY SUFI MASTER

The darkened room is quiet save for a muffled thudding from Tyler's headphones. The boy is so still that his body seems molded into the couch. With his jaw slack and belly distended, Ty's head juts forward in rapt concentration. Light from the TV screen glitters across his eyes. Occasionally he snuffles and clears his throat. Otherwise, nothing moves but his thumbs on the controller.

A voice calls his name and then his mother's body blocks the screen. Craning his neck to see past her, he holds up five fingers. Just then the screen explodes with action and Ty cries out. It's hard to tell if it's an expletive of joy or pain.

Tyler heaves his sixteen-year-old body out of the chair. He rubs at a cramp in his hand and then stretches and yawns. Ambling into the kitchen for a soda, he sullenly picks up the trash can before his mom can say a word. On the back steps, he's ambushed by his kid brother, who wants to shoot some hoops. "Fugeddaboudit," he mutters. Lately, exercise makes his chest hurt. It's been kind of scary.

When he plays video games, Ty holds his breath in reaction to the fantasy crises taking place. When he disappears into that fantasy world, he loses consciousness of his body. The thrill of the game takes his breath away and leaves him drained. He walks with the collapsed posture and shuffling gait of an elderly man.

Many of us—not just teenagers mesmerized by Xbox games—merge with our tasks in a way that mutes self-perception. When we find ourselves in pain or distress, we seldom think that the fault lies in how we have been breathing.

Stopping the World

You may already be aware that you "don't breathe right." Poor breathing habits develop when we misuse the respiratory system to make ourselves feel stable in an unstable world.

Like all living creatures, predators and prey, humans freeze their bodies in response to an emergency. As we strain to catch the next sound or the next glint of light, our stillness stabilizes our eyes and ears for sharp perception and quick reaction. By playing dead we can render ourselves invisible. We also hold our bodies still to restrain anger, block fear, or contain the energy of an overwhelming situation. We hold still to keep emotion from bubbling over and revealing our private selves.

We still our bodies with shallow breathing or by not breathing at all. Although appropriate in a crisis, such "emergency breathing" often overrides the steady ebb and flow of normal respiration. Emergency breathing can become an insidious habit that distorts posture and damages health.

In chapter 2, you learned that your posture zones include structures that lie perpendicular to your body's central axis. When overly constricted, these horizontal stabilizers can close your body around its core. In chapter 3, you experienced improvement to your posture by releasing one of these regions, your pelvic floor. In this chapter, you will explore the horizontally oriented diaphragm. You will see how healthy breathing contributes to open stabilization of your posture and how poor breathing interferes with everything you do or feel.

You may remember Mika from chapter 1, the long-lost friend who moves so fast that her feet barely touch the ground. You don't have to stretch your imagination to see that she's a shallow breather. Her habit of holding her arms tightly to her sides limits her chest's capacity to expand. Her voice has a high, staccato quality and sounds especially strained whenever she raises it. She didn't call out to you, remember? She waited, a little breathlessly, for you to greet her first.

Mika stabilizes her body by making herself small and by never coming to rest. The natural rest that should occur during breathing occurs only when she sighs.

Spiritual teachers of every tradition emphasize the importance of mastering one's breathing as a key to balanced living as well as to achieving higher states of consciousness. Contemporary Westerners take breathing for granted. We are too busy to breathe well. Only when we have some respiratory problem—a head cold or labored breathing from unusual exertion—do we pay much attention to it.

Good—or poor—breathing habits affect every aspect of our bodies' functioning, from our mental state to our digestive efficiency. Breathing is central to our posture and to the way we move. It has huge influence on our appearance, health, mental outlook, emotional resilience, and capacity to manage stress. Dysfunctional breathing is so rampant in Western culture that it amounts to an epidemic.

Take a moment to explore how you breathe. As you remember from chapter 1, trying to observe your breath without controlling it is like trying to lay hands on your shadow. However, the attempt will give you clues about your unconscious habits, and those clues will help you recognize what you're doing in actual circumstances.

Exploration: Quiet Breathing

Rest back into a comfortable chair with your head supported. You should be in a position that is half sitting and half lying down. Rest one hand lightly on your upper chest and the other hand on your lower chest, just above your abdomen.

Breathe in and out in a comfortable, ordinary way. Notice which of your hands moves first when you inhale. This observation indicates your preference for chest or belly breathing.

Now take a deep breath. Which hand moved the most when you took the deeper breath? To breathe deeply, did you use your nose or mouth? These actions indicate your breathing pattern under stress.

Next, while breathing normally, estimate the length of your inhalations and exhalations. Does it take longer to breathe in or out? (Place a clock nearby so that you can count the ticks of the second hand. This is easier than the usual "one one-thousand, two one-thousand" method.)

As you continue breathing comfortably, notice whether there are pauses in your breathing. You may find a pause after inhalation, exhalation, or both.

Describe the effort involved in your inhalation. Does it feel like you are pulling the air inside or does breathing in feel easy, requiring only that you be open to welcome the air?

If your inhalation involves effort, where do you sense it: in your shoulders, neck, chest, or belly?

Now describe the effort of your exhalation. Do you push the air out or simply let it go? Notice whether the outflow of air feels smooth and continuous.

EXPLORATION: ACTIVE BREATHING

For this observation you will need to take a short walk. Notice the features of your breathing while you walk. Do you breathe with your chest, belly, nose, or mouth? Then increase your exertion. Climb some stairs or walk as if you're in a hurry. Describe your breathing under this added stress.

Review these explorations after you have practiced the exercises in this chapter and chapter 5. Give yourself a month or two to make changes and then reassess your breathing.

We'll now explore the mechanics and chemistry of respiration.

THE MECHANICS OF BREATHING

Sensations of breathing are most obvious in the breathing organs—nose, throat, windpipe, and lungs. Most people are also aware of a bellows-like motion within the trunk. When the respiratory muscles contract, they enlarge the rib cage, stretching the lungs and creating a vacuum that draws the air inside. The expansive movement of inhalation alternates with a diminishing action that pushes the air out. Exhalation is caused by the elastic recoil of lung tissue, by the upward movement of the diaphragm as it relaxes, and when the body is upright, by compression of the abdomen.

Because we breathe under all sorts of circumstances and in all sorts of body positions, we need a variety of ways to enlarge the air chamber. We breathe differently at sea level than we do at 14,000 feet, differently while fixing a pipe under the sink than singing around a campfire, and differently still while sprinting for the subway, running a marathon, meditating, or making love. Our bones, muscles, and fascia must adapt to our bodies' changing demands for air just as they do to our constantly changing relationship with gravity. The more active we are, the more we need to enlist accessory

Becoming Lighthearted

Expansion and contraction of your lungs massages your heart as you breathe. At the same time, your diaphragm pulls and pushes on your heart from below, assisting blood flow. When your spine is extended by your use of good breathing mechanics, the fascial envelope around the heart stretches, contributing to the balance of pressures around this essential organ. Healthy posture and breathing actually support your heart. This gives added meaning to the term "lighthearted."

breathing muscles to widen and deepen the rib cage to receive more air. Along with the diaphragm and scalenes described in chapter 1, many other muscles of the chest, shoulders, abdomen, and spine can double as breathing muscles.

There is no single right way to breathe. There are many blends of abdominal and thoracic breathing, but the essential movement of normal respiration is performed by the diaphragm. However, if you receive a blow to your abdomen that immobilizes your diaphragm, you can only gasp for air with your mouth open and shoulders lifted. In such a case your accessory breathing muscles take over.

In chapter 1, we viewed the diaphragm as a dome-shaped muscle whose periphery is fastened around the inside of the lower rib cage. When the diaphragm flattens against the abdomen, it draws the lungs down with it. When the body is at rest, the diaphragm's action pushes the abdomen forward. This "belly breathing" is normal whenever our bodies are supported and relatively inactive. At such times, the diaphragm does 70 to 80 percent of the work of breathing. If you observed your belly moving first during the Quiet Breathing exploration, your passive breathing is as it should be.

Back Support for Inhalation

In addition to its role in breathing that we've already discussed, the diaphragm also has another feature by which it impacts posture. At the back of the diaphragm are some tough muscular fibers that run vertically down the front of the spine from the level of the *solar plexus* to the waist. These muscular fibers, called the *crura,* can operate independently of the dome. Correct function of the crura is essential to healthy breathing, posture, and handling of stress. You can sense the "legs" of the diaphragm tightening behind your abdomen if you bear down as if to defecate. When you do this your belly protrudes and hardens and your back tenses just above your waist. Women naturally use the crura when they engage the diaphragm to push during childbirth.

As you breathe, your diaphragm's motion helps stabilize your trunk by generating pressure within your abdomen. If you sustain a mild bearing-down tension in the crura, you increase the feeling of abdominal stability. Because doing this makes it awkward to use the diaphragm, the habit fosters upper rib cage breathing. Many people misuse the crura in this way when lifting heavy objects, undertaking difficult tasks, or trying to control a situation. Abdominal support is necessary in such circumstances, but crural tension is a poor way to achieve it.

Contraction of both the crura and the scalenes, which are the neck muscles that assist inhalation, pulls the spine forward. To resist this tendency, we must engage our back muscles when we inhale. This means that the natural motion of breathing should include a very slight backward stretch of the spine with inhalation. When we exhale, the spine should relax to its neutral erectness. The resulting subtle articulation of the vertebrae pumps fluid through the vertebral discs, keeping them healthy. Extension of the spine also makes space for the venetian blind–like pivoting of the ribs, which in turn contributes to the lift of the rib cage.

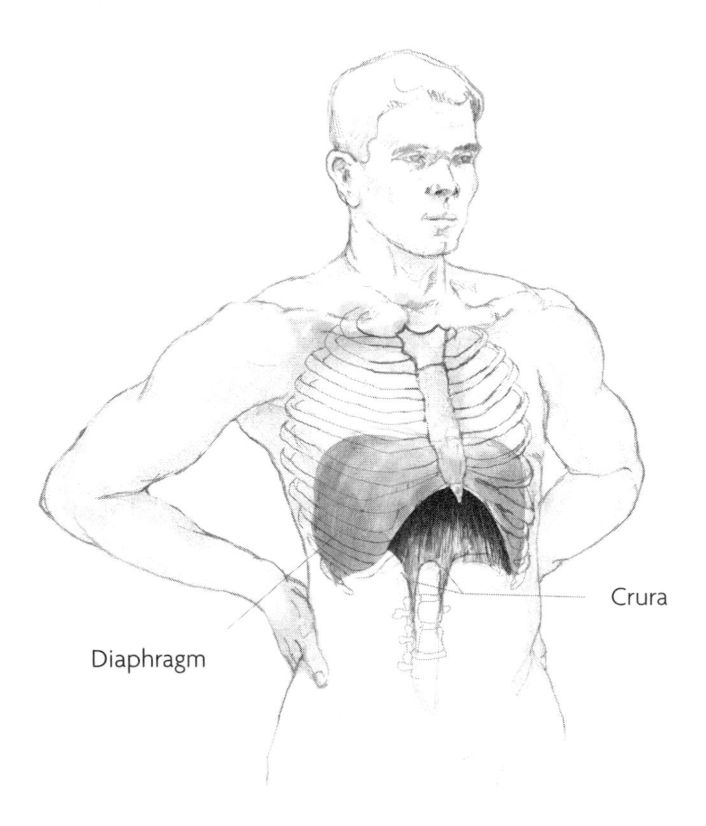

Fig. 4.1. The crura connect the diaphragm to the lumbar spine.

If your spine is stiff with chronic tension, your breathing muscles must work harder to raise your ribs and open your chest. It's a catch-22 situation: learning to breathe well reduces tension along your spine, but to use your breathing muscles efficiently, you need to relax your spine.

When we are at rest, exhalation occurs because the diaphragm relaxes. Exhaling after a belly breath should be a passive event. When we are upright and active, engaging more muscles and taking in more air, the abdominal muscles assist in exhalation. The best muscle for this purpose is the *transversus abdominis,* or *TA,* which wraps around the abdomen like a corset. You can sense the basic activity of your TA with the following experiment.

Standing or sitting with your spine erect, make a polite little cough. Cough as if you were trying to avoid being noticed, without bending forward. You will feel a gentle squeezing of your belly. A slow, steady version of this squeezing action is how exhaling should feel when you are moderately active, as when doing domestic tasks or shopping. You'll explore the transversus abdominis at length in chapter 5.

Nose Power

Your nose is an air conditioner. Spongy bones within each nostril churn the air into thin streams that pass through tiny passages behind your nose. The passages are lined with mucus-producing membranes that adjust the moisture and temperature of the air and microscopic hairs that filter out debris. Your nasal passages do more than condition the air, however. Their resistance to air flow boosts the efficiency of oxygen delivery to your bloodstream. Nose breathing is like putting a nozzle on a garden hose. The same amount of water comes out of the faucet, but the pressure makes the water spray faster and further out into the garden. The nose propels oxygen all the way down into your lower lungs. You can feel this with an experiment.

Take two medium-sized breaths, one each through the nose and mouth. Try to take in the same amount of air each time. Feel the difference in how your body responds.

Nose breathing engages your diaphragm and lower ribs and draws the air deep into your lower lungs, where oxygen absorption is most efficient. Mouth breathing, which activates your upper chest, draws the air into your upper lungs. Extreme breathing that involves the chest, with collarbones and shoulders lifting also, demands extra muscular effort, which raises your heart rate. Blood then rushes so rapidly through the lungs that oxygen delivery is reduced. The result is a vicious circle of faster, shallower, and more effortful breathing along with increasing strain on your heart.

Upper chest breathing is linked with the part of your involuntary nervous system that deals with emergencies, *the sympathetic nervous system.* The sympathetic nervous system primes your body for action by pouring stress hormones such as adrenaline and cortisol into your blood stream. This is healthy only when you really are responding to a crisis and your body uses up the hormones through activity.

Because it takes longer to inhale through your nose than through your mouth, nose breathing automatically slows your breathing down. Exhaling through the nose creates a back pressure that increases the efficiency of oxygen exchange in the lungs. Further, nose breathing is linked to the *parasympathetic system,* the part of your involuntary nervous system that calms your body chemistry, slowing your heart rate, relaxing your muscles, and generally reducing the wear and tear on your body.

Along with its health benefits, nose breathing improves your posture.

This is not as far-fetched as it sounds. When you have correct abdominal support, breathing through your nose expands your lower rib cage. This expansion elongates your trunk and decompresses your lower spine.

People who habitually breathe through their mouths are at a disadvantage in establishing healthy breathing. Mouth breathers often suffer from chronic nasal congestion that makes it difficult for them to breathe through the nose. Excess mucus often can be cleared by two practices borrowed from yoga.

Yoga classes often begin and end by chanting the sound "Om." Research suggests that the "mmmm" sound vibrates the nasal passages and helps them drain. If chanting is not your style, humming any tune can help clear the sinuses.

Many yoga practitioners employ a nasal washing technique called *neti.* The procedure involves pouring warm saline solution into one nostril and letting it drain through the other side. You might expect this to feel as if you had gotten water up your nose while swimming. In fact, as long as you find the right angle to tilt your head while pouring, the process is quite agreeable. Nasal washing is also said to provide relief from sinus infections, colds, and allergies.*

The Buteyko Institute, which offers breathing education for people who have asthma, suggests a third way to clear your nose. First, blow your nose. Then close your nostrils with your fingers and hold your breath for five to ten seconds. Finally, breathe gently through your nose. Repeat until your nose has cleared.†

After you have found a way to eliminate nasal congestion, it may require many months of sincere attention to reestablish the habit of breathing through your nose.

Don't Take a Deep Breath

When someone is in distress, the common advice to breathe deeply will only compound his problem. By inhaling deeply, the person exhales equally deeply, losing too much carbon dioxide and causing the blood to hoard oxygen. The oxygen-starved tissues then trigger more distress.

THE CHEMISTRY OF BREATHING

Although many of us are vaguely aware that we breathe poorly, our problems are not severe enough to make us seek respiratory therapy. We may sometimes get out of breath, but most of the time we take breathing for granted. We may have other complaints, though, such as headaches, muscle aches, cold hands and feet, digestive problems, anxiety, or even chest pain, which we are worried might have something to do with our hearts. All of these symptoms can be caused by deficient blood levels of carbon dioxide.

Wait a minute. Carbon dioxide? We all know that breathing has to do

*Donna Farhi, *The Breathing Book* (New York: Henry Holt and Company, 1996), 64–65.

†Contact information for The Buteyko Institute is found in the appendix.

Backward Breathing

Less common than mouth or upper chest breathing is backward or *paradoxical* breathing, another habit that undermines respiratory efficiency. Paradoxical breathing involves sucking your abdomen in during inhalation and pushing it out during exhalation. You may have noticed yourself doing this in an earlier exercise when you took a deep breath. If not, try it now, just to experience what it feels like to breathe backwards. The habit is common in people who have undergone shock or trauma.

Backward breathing affects body chemistry in a way that perpetuates a feeling of crisis and panic. If this breathing pattern feels familiar, you could benefit from practicing the breathing exercises presented later in this chapter. Should breathing practice make you anxious, however, you may also need to seek trauma counseling.*

*You will find contacts for bodymind approaches to trauma counseling in the appendix.

with taking in oxygen and getting rid of carbon dioxide, so we've probably assumed that oxygen is good and carbon dioxide is bad.

As is usually the case with the body, reality is a little more complex. Carbon dioxide is a byproduct of metabolism, especially of muscular activity. Although it is highly toxic, our bodies need a certain amount to maintain the correct balance of gases in our blood.

If you hold your breath to the breaking point (try it now), what you experience is not a lack of oxygen. In fact, our bodies retain more oxygen than we ordinarily need. What you are feeling is the build-up of carbon dioxide in your bloodstream, which makes your blood too acidic. Your body chemistry makes you crave exhalation to release the excess carbon dioxide.

When you exert yourself, such as when you're shoveling snow, you need more oxygen to fuel yourself. You also produce more carbon dioxide as a byproduct of your activity. The resulting imbalance in your blood chemistry stimulates your brain to call for faster and deeper breathing.

When you're sitting still, you need less oxygen and produce less carbon dioxide. Because your blood chemistry is more stable, your breathing is slow and regular. All too often, however, when minimal exertion is combined with a feeling of urgency, people react by breathing too much. Let's say you're planning a wedding and making a list of everything you will have to attend to: the church, the dress, the invitations, the florist, the caterer, the hotel, the limo—the list goes on.

You can swing from exhilaration to exhaustion in no time because your body responds to mental images of the future as if everything were actually happening right now. You feel breathless because your blood is too acidic, so you start to overbreathe—inhaling and exhaling more. Now you're losing too much carbon dioxide without doing any physical activity to build it up again. By overbreathing, your blood has become too alkaline. This condition, called respiratory alkalosis, can cause everything from depression to low back pain.

Overbreathing, also called hyperventilation, is to air what overeating is to food. When we take in too much of a good thing—more than our bodies can use—we suffer certain consequences. When someone is breathing rapidly under stress, it's easy to recognize acute hyperventilation, but chronic overbreathing often goes undetected. Approximately 10 percent of general medical patients suffer from this problem, which is called chronic hyperventilation syndrome.

Among the many symptoms of hyperventilation are frequent sighing or yawning, breathlessness for no apparent reason, lightheadedness or feeling "spaced out," tingling, numb or cold extremities, aching muscles or joints, heart palpitations, chest pain, upset stomach or irritable bowel syndrome, fatigue, sleeplessness, nightmares, sexual problems, anxiety, and depression. How can all these problems result from overbreathing?

When your blood becomes too alkaline from overbreathing, the part of your nervous system responsible for handling emergencies goes on high alert. Your heart beats faster, adrenaline and other stress chemicals pour into your bloodstream, and your blood pressure rises, muscles tense up, and digestion slows down. These events collect your body's energies for high activity. Your heart's pounding creates a feeling of panic.

When the level of carbon dioxide is low, your body reacts as if it were suffocating. Your blood cells, which have a copious amount of oxygen, stop releasing it to your tissues. This can reduce oxygen delivery to your brain by up to 40 percent. Ironically, by overbreathing, your body becomes starved of oxygen. The sensation of "air hunger" leads to more overbreathing and the perpetuation of the problem.

How Overbreathing Becomes a Habit

Overbreathing is your body's normal reaction to physical or nonphysical stress. It becomes habitual when stress is constant or when features of present stress are similar to those of prior trauma. Even after the original stimulus for hyperventilation has ceased, the habit may be so ingrained that body tissues become acclimated to the alkaline body chemistry. In such a case, overbreathing becomes the body's norm, and its various symptoms become chronic.

Physical causes of hyperventilation include chronic pain, asthma, heart disease, pneumonia, diabetes, fever, prolonged talking, or being at high altitudes. Women commonly experience hyperventilation symptoms during menstruation or pregnancy. Nonphysical causes of hyperventilation include anxiety, depression, perfectionism, loneliness, or any sudden life change such as job loss, divorce, or relocation. Drugs that induce hyperventilation include nicotine, caffeine, and amphetamines.

Note: Hyperventilation is commonly associated with liver or kidney disease. Should you suspect either of these conditions in yourself, you should seek medical treatment along with breathing retraining.

Paradoxically, chronic hyperventilation is commonly caused by the habit of holding the breath. In such a case, holding the breath alternates with over-breathing. You might have this habit if you find yourself frequently sighing or yawning. As mentioned earlier, holding the breath is a way to control the body during emergency.

When breathing stops, the carbon dioxide level in the blood rises because it is not being exhaled. The resulting acidity stimulates more breathing—typically a big sigh or yawn—as a way to rush more oxygen to the brain and tissues and to push carbon dioxide levels down. However, inhaling more means you are exhaling more as well, thus, your blood chemistry vacillates between being too acidic and too alkaline.

We hold our breath because it works. It stops the world, momentarily. We might be nervous about taking an exam, for example—a first driving test or the law boards. We might be frustrated while threading a needle by our failing eyesight. We might be stifling anger about a friend's betrayal. Concentration, searching the memory, and indecision all trigger a need to feel stable, but stopping our breathing can never help us think or perceive clearly. In fact, because we are getting less blood to the brain, the result is quite the opposite. Also, if we have adopted "emergency breathing" for too many minor emergencies, the habit can alter the body's chemistry.

Recall Tyler, the teenager who is lost in a video world. His emergencies are imaginary, but his body reacts as if the games were real. Stress hormones flood his bloodstream, readying his body for action, but the only movement he makes is with his thumbs on the controller. The habit of holding his breath has tightened his chest muscles and diaphragm, so when he tries to play basketball his chest hurts, a symptom he's afraid to talk about. The real world of mom and kid brother becomes a burden.

Restoring Healthy Breathing

To restore healthy posture, you must teach yourself to breathe well. This involves both general relaxation of your body and cultivation of specific breathing sensations. It also involves commitment to breathing practice over the long haul. Breathing, our most deeply embedded habit, takes time to change. Five minutes of twice-daily practice for three to six months is a realistic estimate.

The right way to breathe depends on what you're doing. When you're lying down, belly breathing is normal. Under extreme duress, chest breathing may be your only choice. If you're running a marathon, you need a combination of chest and belly breathing. For normal breathing under ordinary circumstances—sitting at work, driving, or walking across the parking lot—breathing should be slow, smooth, and constant, moderate in the amount of air taken in, and involve three-dimensional movement in the rib cage. The exercises that follow foster these features of healthy breathing.

If the breathing center in your brain has reset to accommodate imbalanced blood chemistry, breathing practice to change that can trigger feelings of air hunger. Should this happen during your practice, remember that you feel the urge to breathe because you are accumulating the right amount of carbon dioxide in your blood, not because you don't have enough oxygen. Your air hunger is actually a good sign, indicating that your tissues are trying to return to normal carbon dioxide levels. If you feel the urge to yawn, interrupt it by swallowing. You must then resist the urge to take a deep breath. As you practice moderate breathing, your body will gradually become accustomed to taking in less air.

You will do the first several breathing practices lying down so that you can explore your breath without having to contend with gravity. You will need a towel or blanket folded lengthwise to make a pad about two inches thick and slightly narrower than the width of your back. This pad has three functions: it will support your lumbar curve, open your front ribs, and help you sense your breathing in the back of your rib cage.

Seat yourself on the floor (carpeted and warm, so you can relax) with your buttocks just in front of your blanket. Then lie back over the pad so that everything from your waist up is supported by it. Place a folded towel under your head and neck to raise your head slightly higher than your chest and insure an open airway. Loosen your clothing, especially belts and bras. We become accustomed to belts and bras and don't realize the extent to which they restrict the movement of the diaphragm and lower ribs. Many people find that just resting in this position makes breathing feel easier and more complete.

The more you can allow gravity to support your body, the easier it is to breathe with your diaphragm. Look for a gentle swelling and settling of your belly without forcing it to happen.

If you have become accustomed to upper chest breathing or if you breathe paradoxically (see box on p. 74), relearning the sensations of diaphragmatic breathing may make you feel frustrated or anxious. If this is true for you, try rolling over onto one side. You may find it easier to sense the movement of your diaphragm and belly while lying curled up. Prop

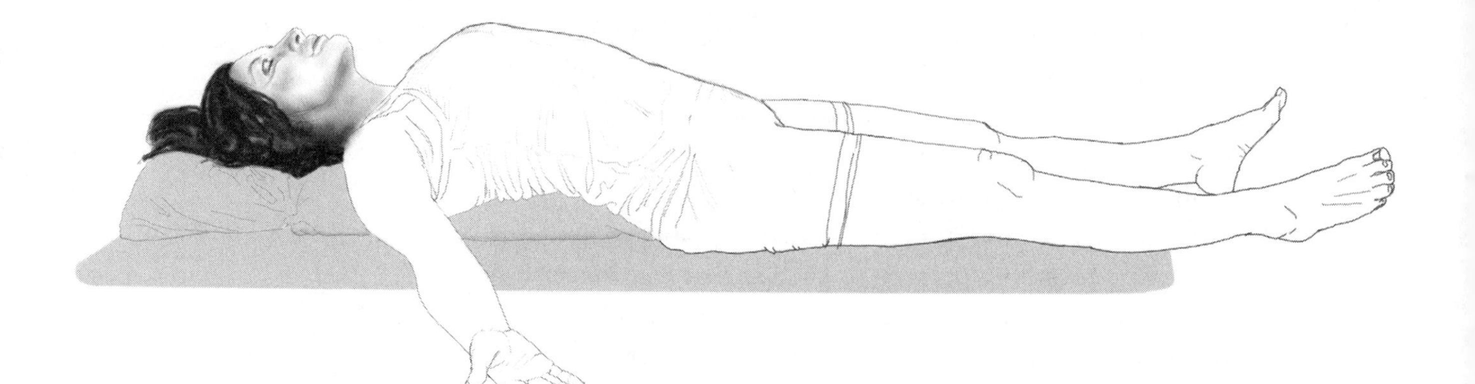

Fig. 4.2. Supported lying position for breathing practices.

yourself comfortably with cushions so you can feel supported while you focus on softening your abdomen. Take all the time you need to restore your belly breathing—days or even weeks—before attempting the other breathing practices.

Practice: Global Breathing Awareness

Begin by simply noticing your body's sensations as you breathe in and out through your nose. As you breathe in, notice an opening sensation, as if breathing has increased the interior space of your body. Feel your inhalation expand the surface area of your skin. As you exhale, feel how your body shrinks and settles. Because your lungs and breathing muscles have fascial connections to every other part of your body, the expansion and contraction of breathing occurs everywhere. Your forearms, fingers, neck, thighs, and ankles all swell and shrink.

If you think you're imagining this phenomenon, test it by doing the opposite: try to feel your body diminishing in size as you inhale and swelling up as you exhale.

Three-Dimensional Breath

Many people move only the front of the rib cage when they breathe. To fully engage the lungs, breathing should expand the ribs to the sides and back as well as front. Expanding only in front also shortens and tightens muscles along the spine. This tension draws your posture back onto your heels and orients your stance behind the gravitational axis. If you felt, during the Global Breathing Awareness practice, that breathing took place mostly in the front of your ribs, use the following exercise to cultivate the motion of breathing that includes the sides and back of your rib cage.

Practice : Breathing in Your Back

Kneel on a soft carpet or exercise mat with your shins forming a "V"—big toes together and knees apart. Bend forward at the hips and rest your forehead on the floor. Rest your arms wherever they are comfortable. If the position strains your knees, place a bolster on your legs and then rest your head and chest on the bolster. You can also do this practice while seated in a chair with your head resting on a table.

Take time to settle into the position. Relax your neck to let the weight of your head rest fully into the floor or cushion. Soften any tension in your abdomen, hips, or legs.

Now breathe into the sides of your lower rib cage. Continue this until it feels easy. Then notice how the sideways motion opens your rib cage to the back. Feel the ribs in your lower back rising toward the ceiling each time you inhale.

Try to sustain the sensations of breathing in your back ribs when you are lying on your back. Inhale down into the floor while simultaneously letting your ribs expand to front and sides. The movement of your breath should be three-dimensional.

The Vacation Within Your Breath

Experts suggest that normal resting respiration should occur at a rate of ten to fourteen breaths per minute. Men tend to breathe more slowly than women. For a rate of twelve breaths per minute, a good breakdown would be inhalation for two seconds, exhalation for three seconds, and a pause of one second. As you begin breathing practice, what's important is not strict adherence to this ratio but rather a sense of similar proportions. Exhalation should take longer than inhalation and should be followed by a pause.

The pause is the completion of exhalation and a vacation before beginning the next breathing cycle. This gives your diaphragm a rest and, because your heart rate automatically slows during exhalation, the pause also rests your heart. Further, the pause lets your blood chemistry signal the respiratory center in your brain that it's time to inhale again.

The next several breathing practices will help you find a healthy balance between inhalation, exhalation, and the respiratory pause. They also will help you slow your breathing down. Breathing slowly checks the habit of breathing too much.

Body-Mind Connections

As modern Westerners, we commonly speak of needing "breathing room." The correlation of breathing with personal space is in accordance with physiological reality. If the air cells *(alveoli)* within our lungs were dissected and spread out flat, their surface area would be about the size of a large living room. When we make full use of the space within our lungs, our posture automatically improves. Having a more erect spine and a more open rib cage correlates with positive, spacious perceptions of ourselves.

The act of breathing is symbolic. Opening our bodies to receive the breath represents our openness to the world of things and other people. The outbreath symbolizes our release of the outside world and return to the home within ourselves.

Practice: Inhaling Beauty

Resting back over your folded blanket, remind yourself of an aroma that gives you pleasure. Inhaling through your nose, imagine that you are smelling a lovely rose or delicious fresh-baked cookies. Take in a moderate amount of air. Feel your nostrils widening all the way back to the depths of your nostrils. Let the scent flow in along with feelings of receptivity and gratitude.

If you find it difficult to imagine an aroma, picture a beautiful scene, with light and color that bring you pleasure. Inhale while opening yourself to that space. Invite the space to enter your body.

The Inhaling Beauty practice helps you develop full use of your diaphragm and rib cage. The visualization tricks your nervous system into producing an easy inhalation. If it feels hard to do this with every inhalation, take a few ordinary breaths between tries.

Practice: Exhaling Surrender

As you breathe out through your nose, turn your attention to the weight of your body on the floor. Rather than focusing directly on exhalation, concentrate on the sensation of your body's weightedness. During each exhalation, choose a body part to sense—ankles, hips, fingers, elbows, jaw, eyes, intestines, or liver. The choices are nearly limitless. Discover which part of your body rests most easily into the floor. Savor that sensation and then let the feeling spread to parts of your body that seem less weighted. With each exhalation, deepen your body's surrender to gravity. Gradually let all parts of your body match the heaviness of the heaviest part.

By relaxing your body in this way, you also relax the muscles of inhalation. Relaxing your diaphragm is essential to full exhalation. You will find that this practice slows down your exhalation and lengthens the pause at its end. Inhaling will also feel increasingly automatic, effortless, and pleasurable.

This practice induces deep relaxation, so take time to restore your awareness of your surroundings when you are finished. Open your eyes, roll onto one side, and gently push yourself up to a sitting position.

Practice: The Spaciousness and Weight of Breathing

When you feel comfortable with the Inhaling Beauty and Exhaling Surrender practices, you can combine them into a single breathing exercise. On every second or third breath, open your body to receive the outside space as you inhale and then release your body's weight to the earth as you exhale. Between attempts, breathe through your nose in an ordinary way. Always inhale moderately rather than deeply, and remember to let your ribs expand to the sides and back as well as in front.

The practices Inhaling Beauty and Exhaling Surrender help you savor the sensations of breathing. As you cycle between sensations of lightness and weightedness, fullness and emptiness, and swelling and shrinking, your body will release the hidden tensions that have prevented your breathing from being complete.

Practice: Breathing in Gravity

When this supported practice feels easy, you can graduate to seated breathing practice. Recall the features of healthy sitting. Make sure that your pelvic floor diamond is spacious and your lumbar spine has a neutral forward curve. Let your shoulder blades rest on the back of your rib cage and your collarbones broaden. The way you are sitting should make it easy for your rib cage to expand to the sides and back as well as in front.

As you inhale, open your body to take in the space from outside yourself. Let your body welcome the air so that your breath can occur without effort. When you breathe out, be aware of support from the floor, the chair seat, and your own spine. Sense the weight of your body without letting your spine or chest collapse. Let each inward breath arise naturally from the pause at the end of each outward breath. Breathe at a slow and constant rate and take in moderate amounts of air. Because you are at rest, there's no need for inhalation to expand fully into your upper ribs. Lower rib cage breathing is all you need.

When seated breathing practice feels easy, begin attending to your breathing during daily activities. Choose moments such as waiting on the phone or sitting at red lights.

Mika Waits to Exhale

At first Mika hated breathing practice. It made her antsy, but she had a hunch that breathing was the key to her bouts of anxiety. The only time she ever got a full breath was when she took a drag on a cigarette.

One night, when her neighbor came over to watch a video, she had an inspiration. Alfredo was always ready for something new. "Here," she said, "read these instructions to me so I can relax."

Soon Alfredo and Mika set up a buddy system to notice when they held their breath or sped it up. They challenged themselves by checking their breathing during the slasher movies they both loved.

For Mika, the feeling of weightedness was the elusive thing. She couldn't seem to stay comfortable inside her own skin long enough to let the pause occur.

"You never pause," Alfredo told her. "Even during the movie you're popping up to fix snacks or tidy the kitchen. C'mon," he said, "give yourself a breather."

GETTING IT RIGHT

During breathing practice, be sure that you do not take in more air than you need as you attempt to slow your exhalation. The whole point is lost if you overbreathe. Dysfunctional breathing patterns are often linked to perfectionism, so, if you approach breathing practice with the wish to get it right immediately, you'll narrow your chance of success. Changing your breathing requires patience, persistence, and respect for your body's capacity to change at its own pace.

If you have a history of allergies or asthma and have developed habitual mouth and upper chest breathing, changing your breathing habits will take many months of dedicated practice. If it's not comfortable to slow every breath, do so every third breath, or every fifth. Whatever you can do to begin changing your breathing pattern will be a good start.

Practice: Slowing Your Breath with Sound

A sounding technique used in yoga called *ujjahi* breathing will help you slow your breathing. After a moderate inhalation, imagine saying "Ahhh" as you exhale with your mouth closed. Your imagined vocalization causes a slight narrowing of your throat and a soft hissing sound as if there were a distant wind inside your body. The "Ahhhs" should be just loud enough for you to monitor the pace, evenness, and ease of your breath. Avoid exhaling beyond your ability to make the sound easily.

Using sound is an exercise to slow your breathing. Be sure also to practice without sounding so that tension in your throat does not become a habit. In daily life, your throat should be soft and open when you breathe.

As you make the "Ahhh" sound during exhalation, you will feel a subtle squeezing sensation across your lower abdomen. This is the action of your transversus abdominis, the correct muscle to use during exhalation. Practicing this will prepare you for the exploration of abdominal support in the next chapter.

Practice: Healthy Breathing, Healthy Posture

Healthy breathing fosters healthy posture and graceful movement. This practice helps you feel this for yourself. As you lie in the supported breathing position, take a few minutes to review your breathing practice. While doing so, enjoy the openness of your chest, the breadth of your collarbones, and the release of your shoulder blades back onto the floor. Relax your buttocks and allow your pelvic floor to be spacious. Soften your jaw and throat. As you exhale, appreciate the luxury of resting your body into the floor. Now, take several moments to picture yourself standing up while sustaining these sensations of healthy breathing. Then roll to one side and bring yourself up to a standing position.

If you have done this practice with patience and care, you will likely find yourself standing taller than usual. You may also feel that your feet are more securely planted on the ground. In addition to removing tensions that prevent good posture, breathing well also stimulates positive tensions that are needed to support good posture.

Take a short walk to notice how it feels to move. When better breathing improves your posture, your better posture makes movement feel more fluid.

Eating Practice

Mouth breathers tend to inhale while eating or drinking. If you notice yourself gulping air along with your orange juice, you need to set aside some mealtimes during which you pay attention to breathing. Open your mouth to eat or drink during the pause after an exhalation. Inhale after you've swallowed the liquid. Eating practice will slow down your eating as well as your breathing. The cultivation of relaxed eating habits interrupts the habit of overbreathing and contributes to better digestion as well.

Elevation of your rib cage gives support to your shoulders, neck, and head. Reduced shoulder tension contributes to freer movement of your arms. The relaxed arm swing helps generate freer hip and leg movement.

Breathing and Stability

We ruin our breathing when we misuse it to control situations or to stifle emotions. Although our bodies require stabilization under duress, most of us do this in the wrong ways. We try to secure our bodies with our breathing muscles because we've forgotten how to correctly support and contain ourselves with our abdominal muscles. This is the topic of chapter 5.

All of the characters you've met in this book will be grateful for the next chapter. Alison, who holds her breath when she concentrates; Carmen, who has back pain despite her dedication to crunches at the gym; and slender Mika, who is always complaining about the potbelly she can't get rid of. Each of them will discover that life becomes more manageable when they discover the secret of internal support. As for Tyler, the teenager on the couch, perhaps a miracle. . . .

5 CORE CONNECTIONS

> *Those who would preserve the spirit must also look after the body to which it is attached.*
>
> ALBERT EINSTEIN

Broad-shouldered, muscular, and good-looking, Nick doesn't seem like someone who suffers from chronic back pain. But you can see it when he walks. It looks as though getting from one foot to the other costs him more than it should. In fact, searing pain makes him catch his breath four or five times a day. He's thirty-two.

Nick grew up snowboarding and mountain biking in Colorado. From the time he could walk, he was out taking chances and taking spills. By the time he entered college, he'd undergone two knee surgeries. Two rounds of physical therapy helped him rebuild strength in his legs, but Nick still didn't feel steady on his feet. Unconsciously, he clenched his buttock muscles to center himself and tensed his shoulders to hoist his weight up off his knees. These habits made him walk with a rolling gait that the neighbor kids thought looked cool.

After college, Nick went to work in an office. He was glad to be paying off his student loans, but he hated being stuck indoors and sitting all day made his back stiff. On weekends, he enrolled in a program to become an emergency medical technician. Always cool under pressure, he knew that he had a good head for search and rescue. The work combined problem solving and service, and he felt he'd found his calling—no more penance behind a desk.

However, one day it was Nick being carried out on a litter. He'd done nothing special, just a little twist when a rock shifted underfoot. Afterward he couldn't stand up. A disc between two lumbar vertebrae had ruptured.

It's been five years and two back surgeries since that turn in the mountains. After the first surgery, Nick strapped on a backpack way too soon and found himself back in the hospital. Now his doctor wants to fuse the vertebrae, but Nick's experience tells him surgery holds no guarantees. He's decided to try improving his back with exercise.

All of Nick's physical therapists have told him he needs strong abdominal muscles to stabilize his spine. A girlfriend who took some Pilates lessons showed him how to do half sit-ups, flattening his back against the floor while he lifts his chest and head. Doing this a hundred times every day makes his abdominal muscles feel taut, but his back still aches much of the time. Nick longs to get back on the trail, but the heavy gear required in search and rescue work aggravates his back even though he can do more sit-ups and push-ups than ever before. Nick worries that he's chained to a desk after all.

His therapists are right about Nick's spine needing support—experts in physical medicine have long recognized the link between faulty spinal stabilization and low back pain.

Unlike the solid vertical beams of a building, the vertical support of the body is segmented. The spine has separate, distinct vertebrae, each having many joints. This feature of human structure is at the core of the negotiation between our need to stabilize our bodies and our need to move. When loads are placed on the spine—whether heavy paramedic equipment or a tired toddler—the joints between the vertebrae must be held stable enough for the trunk to sustain the extra weight. This is what Nick has been trying to do—stabilize his back so that he can carry heavy loads and walk.

The problem is that Nick is achieving stability in the wrong ways. He tucks his tail down, believing that his lower back should be flat. Because he's training his pelvis in a backward tilt, he assumes he should sit and walk with a flat spine as well. In so doing, he sabotages his spine's natural spring system and puts more pressure on the injured disc.

Second, the way he's been taught to strengthen his abdominal muscles actually weakens the muscles that should be giving him the deepest support. To understand this, we need to be clear about the anatomy of the abdomen. Fitness professionals and physical therapists commonly refer to this area as "the core."

What Is the Core?

"Core" has become a buzzword. A Google search yields millions of web pages that tout strengthening exercises and fitness equipment. However, many of these programs simply use the term "core" to mean the abdominal muscles—the "abs." To fully understand the nature of healthy posture, we need a deeper sense of what the core really is.

Strictly speaking, the core of something is its most central and essential part. In the case of your body, the true core is the site of your internal organs. These organs, consisting of up to 90 percent water, are contained within a bag of fascia called the *peritoneum*. You can picture the peritoneum as an elongated water balloon suspended from the inside surface of your back.

The back wall of the balloon is protected and supported by the spine and the back of the pelvis. However, the front of your body is soft so that it can adapt to the organs as they undergo mundane events such as the movement of toxic gases after a bout of overeating or awesome events such as pregnancy and delivery. Containing and protecting the organs are several layers of muscle that crisscross the abdomen like a girdle. Their contraction stabilizes the internal organs by increasing pressure within the abdomen. Fitness professionals call these muscles the "core."

The core muscles form two corsets—an inner one that has direct connections to the spine and a more superficial outer one that does not. Healthy posture depends on your being able to distinguish between these two very different types of core muscle support.

Anatomy: The Inner Corset

The main muscle of the inner corset is the transversus abdominis, or the TA, which you already learned about in connection with exhalation. The TA is a broad, horizontal sheet that wraps around the visceral core. In front, it blends into a layer of fascia that runs between the breastbone and the pubic bone. In back, its fibers attach to the upper rim of the pelvis, the fascia of the lumbar spine, and the inside surface of the lower ribs.

Contraction of the TA compresses the abdomen and tightens the lumbar fascia. Although the muscle extends as far up as the diaphragm, it is the contraction of the lower fibers—between pubic bone and navel—that is crucial for lower back stability. The TA squeezes, but does not bend, twist, or tilt the trunk. This distinguishes it from the muscles of the outer corset.

Women's Issues

Women have special needs for a healthy approach to core support because women's bodies are naturally more prone than men's to fluctuations of weight and pressure in the abdomen and pelvis. From the monthly menstrual cycle to pregnancy and menopause, women's bodies are continually bombarded by their hormones. Many women respond to hormonal fluctuations by developing chronic tension in the wrong abdominal corset. They pinch themselves in at the waist, trying to look thin. The result is that millions of women suffer unnecessarily from poor breathing habits, reduced sexual responsiveness, and urinary incontinence.

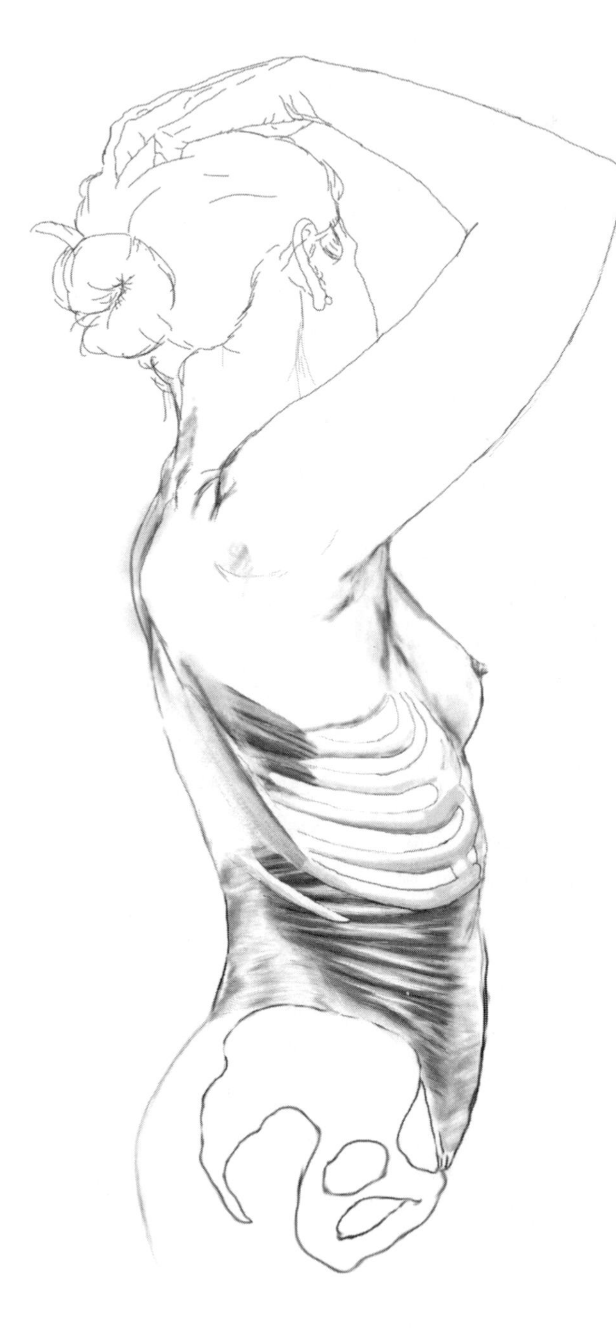

Fig. 5.1. The transversus abdominis muscle wraps from front to back, where it connects with the multifidi. This is the inner corset.

The way the TA blends into the lumbar fascia is key to its role in stabilizing the lower back. Within the lumbar fascia on both sides of the spine are five muscle bundles called the *multifidi* that run between individual lumbar vertebrae. When the TA activates the lumbar fascia, the multifidi are stimulated to control the lumbar segments. This means that although the TA is a broad expanse of muscle, its action on the lumbar spine is very specific. Studies show that the TA contracts to stabilize your body before you use your arms or legs.

For example, let's say you've been asked a question by a teacher in school. You raise your hand, eager to be the first to give the right answer. Try this now: raise your hand with a lot of enthusiasm. As your arm went up, you probably took a quick inhalation. In part, the diaphragm's action prepares you for speech, but it also contributes pressure within your abdomen to help stabilize your trunk. This pressure should be met by matching pressure from the TA.

Studies have shown that the TA is active prior to contraction of arm or leg muscles only in people who have no history of low back pain.* This indicates a direct link between the health of the inner corset and a healthy spine. This deep core musculature also supports the rotary movements of the lumbar spine that are essential to healthy walking. Inner corset activity is what Nick's rehab program failed to address.

Anatomy: The Outer Corset

One of the outer corset muscles runs vertically from breastbone to pubic bone. Others run diagonally and crisscross the abdomen between the front of the lower

*Carolyn Richardson et al., *Therapeutic Exercise for Spinal Segmental Stabilization in Low Back Pain* (Edinburgh: Churchill Livingstone, 1999), 61–63.

rib cage and the groin. Together, these muscles act to bend your trunk forward and twist it to either side. Although the outer corset muscles contribute to generalized trunk stability, they are not attached to the spine and therefore can't give it direct support. In fact, if the outer corset muscles become overly short and tight, they draw the chest and pelvis together which flattens the lumbar spine. This puts excessive pressure on the lumbar discs. Downward drag on your rib cage also restricts your diaphragm and leads to upper chest breathing. Further, a shortened outer corset makes your back muscles overwork to keep you upright. In short, excessive stabilization by the outer corset compresses your core and closes your posture.

To become aware of your outer corset, lie on your back and contract your abdominal muscles in a way that flattens your back to the floor and draws your lower ribs down and together in front. Notice how this action restricts your breathing.

Make the same abdominal contraction while standing up. The action will tuck your tail under and compress your chest. Walk around while maintaining outer corset tension and notice how it blocks freedom of movement in your whole body. You can't breathe freely, and with your pelvis tucked under, you can't freely move your legs.

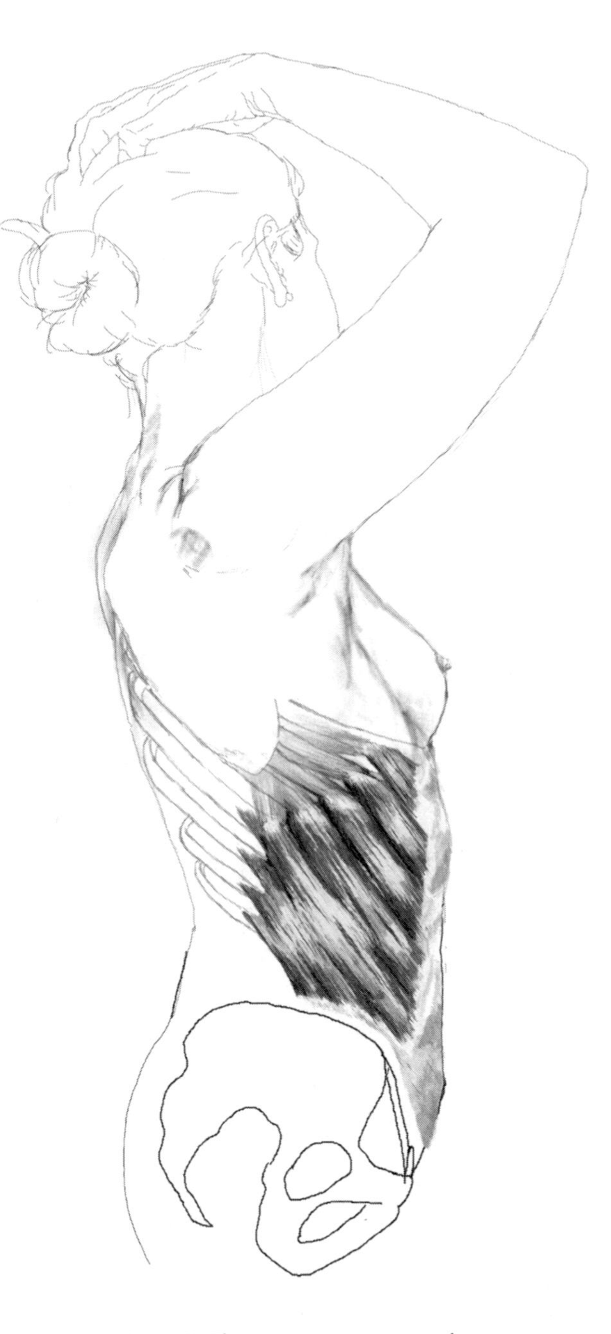

Fig. 5.2. The outer corset muscles, including the *external abdominal obliques* shown here, connect the pelvis and the rib cage. Because they are not attached to the spine, they cannot support it directly.

The Core and Lower Back Pain

Practitioners of physical medicine have long recognized the need for abdominal support for the spine. However, as Nick discovered, just strengthening the abs does not accomplish the desired result. Research suggests that the secret to prevention and elimination of low back pain is sustained contraction of the TA.*

---

*Carolyn Richardson et al., *Therapeutic Exercise for Spinal Segmental Stabilization in Low Back Pain* (Edinburgh: Churchill Livingstone, 1999), 48–49.

In fact, just 10 to 25 percent of your perceived maximum effort is sufficient to support the lower back and prevent problems from developing. This means that for healthy posture the muscle should be mildly active whenever your body is upright and moving, but TA contraction can be difficult to feel because it does not entail overt movement. In fast-paced exercise classes, teachers don't have time to teach the subtle sensations involved in strengthening the inner corset.

Most fitness and rehabilitation programs that promote core strengthening overemphasize the outer corset muscles, which are easy to sense because they cause bodily movement. That makes strengthening them easy to teach. When you do a sit-up, you can see and feel yourself moving. However, outer corset emphasis can actually overwhelm the inner corset and make it weaker. This is what was happening to Nick. Because of his dedication to strengthening his abs, the muscles most equipped to support his beleaguered spine were actually getting weaker. A detour into muscle physiology will explain why this was happening.

Muscles are composed of millions of threadlike cells or fibers. The fibers are of two types: some are good for feats of strength or bursts of activity and others can hold muscle tension in a steady state. Physiologists call the fibers "fast twitch" and "slow twitch" fibers, respectively. Fast twitch fibers contract rapidly and tire rapidly. Slow twitch fibers sustain continuous or repeated contractions, such as those made by the diaphragm, without tiring.

Most muscles contain fibers of both types. A muscle develops more of one type or the other depending on how it's being used. Muscles responsible for maintaining posture develop more endurance, or slow twitch, fibers.

In the abdomen, the outer corset muscles have mostly speed and strength fibers, and the inner corset muscles have mostly endurance fibers. However, if the TA is underactive for some reason—let's say it was cut during surgery or stretched too far during childbirth—it loses integrity. During sit-ups, the TA's fast twitch fibers contract along with the outer corset muscles. In this way, the TA loses its capacity to contract slowly and sustain tension. It is as if it has forgotten how to do its real job.

If you have an underactive TA, standard abdominal exercises will not engage it and will, in fact, override it. Core strengthening programs are successful only if you can distinguish the subtle sensation of TA activity clearly enough to be sure you are using it.

In chapter 4, you explored the TA in connection with breathing. Remind yourself of the feeling of the "polite cough," in which you compressed your abdomen without bending forward. The practices in this section will help you develop a mild, sustained version of that sensation. Four different inner corset exercises follow. Because the feeling of TA contraction can be elusive, some of you will find it easier to access in one way more than another. Practice the exercises that make the sensations clearest for you.

Each practice begins by establishing your spine's natural lumbar curve. The curve should not change when you engage your TA. If your lumbar curve flattens when you do the exercises, it will mean that you are using your outer corset muscles.

After you've engaged your inner corset, your challenge will be to breathe naturally while sustaining the contraction. If your TA is underactive, this may be harder than it sounds. Developing your inner corset requires attention rather than effort and a willingness to be interested in your body's internal sensations.

While you're learning to engage your TA, you should stop doing ab-strengthening workouts such as sit-ups or the Pilates Hundred exercise. Such exercises engage the outer corset by calling for rapid movements. To recognize the sensations of inner corset activity, your outer corset must be relaxed. If you are physically fit, this may be difficult because your TA has been overpowered by the outer muscles. After you have mastered TA engagement, you can return to your usual routine, incorporating your new skill.

If your inner corset is underactive, you'll need several months of practice before you can call the TA your own. Luckily, when you've found the right sensation, you can practice while you're doing other things. Your goal should be for the sensation of inner corset support to become so familiar that you'll habitually access it whenever you are upright.

Practice: Activating Your TA through the Pelvic Floor

This practice is an indirect route to sensing your inner corset. For many people, it is the easiest way to feel the TA working. The exercise takes advantage of the fascial continuity between muscles of the pelvic floor and the TA.

The bottom of your core is contained and supported by the perineum, the muscular hammock that spans your pelvic floor diamond. When you contract the front triangle of the perineum, you will activate the lower fibers of the TA as well.

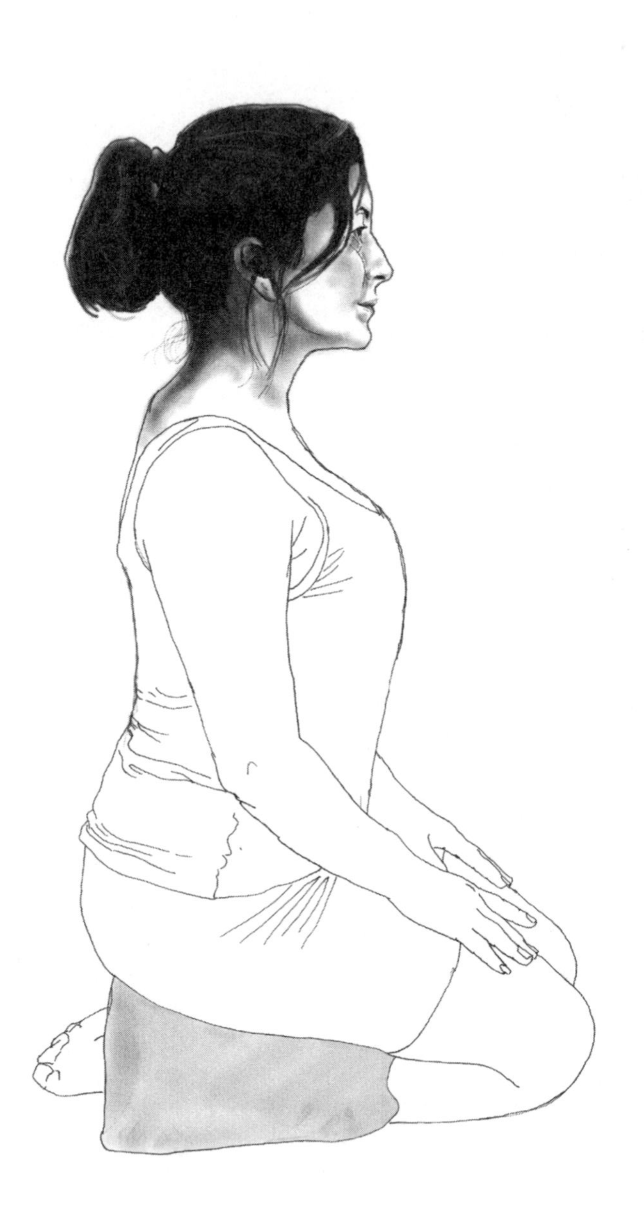

Fig. 5.3. Kneeling position for engaging the pelvic floor muscles.

To begin, kneel on a padded surface and sit on your heels. If kneeling strains your knees, place a cushion between your thighs and buttocks and sit on the cushion. If the position strains your ankles and feet, place a rolled towel under your ankles. The kneeling position allows you to use your own legs for feedback about doing the practice correctly. If nothing you do makes kneeling comfortable, you can do this exercise while sitting on a chair.

Sit on your heels with a neutral lumbar curve, your back triangle relaxed, and your chest lifted. Relax the abdominal muscles. Establish slow, moderate breathing through your nose. Feel the lower ribs expanding to the front, sides, and back as you breathe with your diaphragm.

Before taking your next inhalation, gradually contract your perineal muscles as if trying not to urinate. Maintain that contraction and resume breathing. After two or three breath cycles, relax your pelvic floor and rest.

Notice whether you felt your weight dropping onto your legs when you relaxed. If you did, you were not isolating the action of the perineal muscles. Instead, you were engaging muscles of your buttocks and thighs along with those of the pelvic floor. Try again. After an exhalation, draw up slowly through your perineum. This time avoid lifting your pelvis up from your legs. Concentrate on contracting the urogenital or front triangle. The sensation will be a mild retraction of the clitoris for women, and of the penis for men. The front of the perineum has fascial connections to the part of the TA that you're trying to access. While it's easier to contract the anal triangle, doing so tends to tuck the coccyx under and flatten the lumbar curve.

The contraction should not produce any backward pelvic tilt or change in the position of your spine. Nothing should happen except within the core of your body, a sensation you will likely sense as a centralized lift. You should feel a mild shrinking of the tissues across your lower abdomen—below your navel—and mild activity in your lumbar muscles, as if they were very subtly filling out.

If you're not sure what you feel, use your hands for feedback. Place one hand across your abdomen below your navel. Rest it there as lightly as a napkin on your lap. When you perform your next perineum contraction, feel your abdomen drawing away from your hand. Rest your other hand behind your back, with the back of your hand against your lower spine. With the next contraction, sense the subtle swelling of your multifidi muscles against the back of your hand.

This practice engages your pelvic floor muscles to help you activate your TA. This does not mean that you should strive to maintain constant contraction of your pelvic floor. To the contrary, you should be able to activate your TA independently of your perineum. The next practices help you do this.

The Original Kegel Exercise

Women readers will be familiar with this perineum exercise as a means to enhance sexual functioning and restore urinary control after tissue damage during childbirth. In the 1960s, Arnold Kegel, M.D., was the first to teach women to strengthen the perineum by interrupting urinary flow—urinating a spoonful at a time. The exercise is a good way to strengthen your perineum and engage your inner corset as well. What is different in the healthy posture version is the emphasis on contracting the front of the perineum—the urogenital triangle—rather than tightening your buttocks or tucking your tail.

Practice: Activating Your TA from a Table Position

Establishing a neutral position of your spine is critical for the success of this practice, so have patience with the details of the starting position. You will need to work on a carpeted surface. Position yourself on hands and knees, placing a rolled towel under your ankles if they are stiff. Line up your limbs so that your wrists are directly beneath your armpits and your knees are directly below your hip creases. Relax your hips so that your pelvic floor diamond is spacious. The position should establish a gentle sway in your lumbar spine. If it makes your derriere seem vulnerable, you've probably got it right.

Open your hands to allow space between your fingers and rotate your upper arms so that the creases of your elbows face forward. Then, draw your shoulder blades toward your sacrum and press your palms and fingers into the floor. These actions should broaden your upper back and open your chest—all without changing your lumbar curve or tilting your pelvis under. To put a gentle curve in your neck, gaze at the floor about twelve inches in front of your hands. You've now established a neutral position for your spine. Let your abdomen relax completely; feel it hanging from your spine.

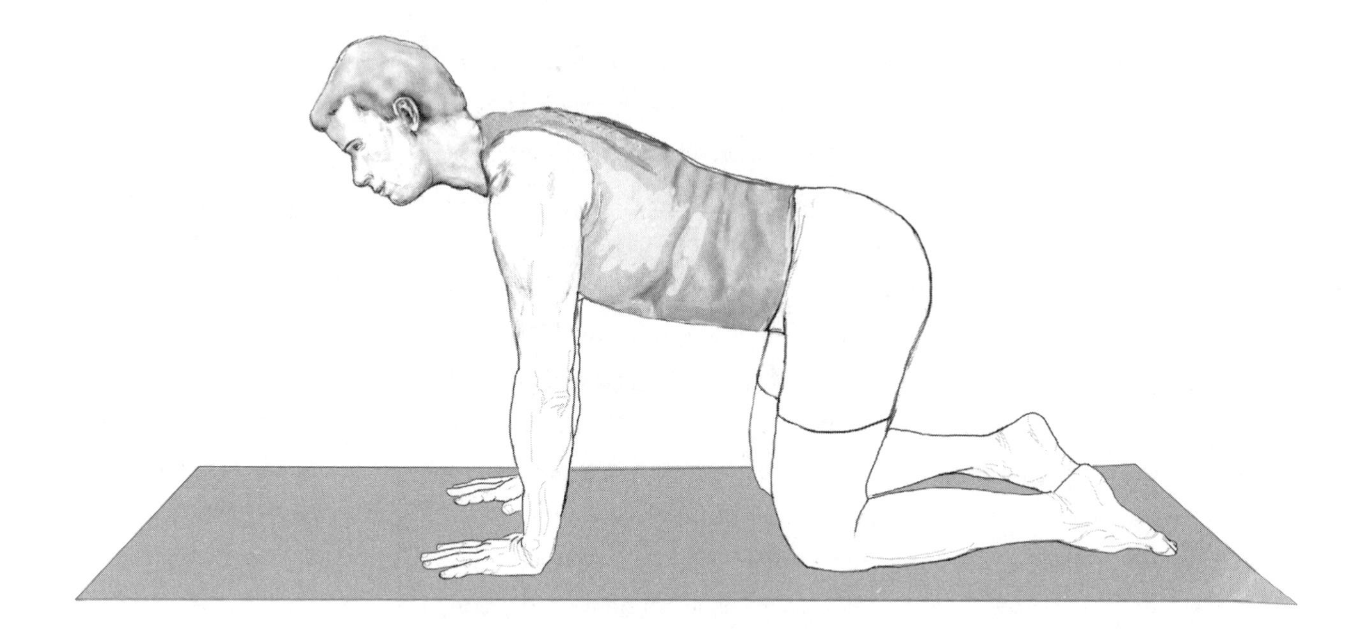

Fig. 5.4. Table position for activating your TA.

Breathe slowly and moderately through your nose. Feel your breath filling both the front and back of your rib cage. Feel it widening your lower ribs. Inhale again, exhale, and then, without taking in another breath, very slowly and gradually draw your lower abdomen in and up, away from the ground.

Focus your attention on the part of your abdomen that lies between your pubic bone and navel. Imagine that you are wearing a bikini and that the front of it is shrinking. Alternatively, imagine your intestines sliding in and up toward the back of your waist, as if you were "swallowing" them upward.

Along with the sensation of your abdomen rising, look for accompanying activity in your lumbar muscles. This should be a faint sensation of activity in your lower back but not a movement of your spine. You may not feel it immediately, but if you persist, the TA sensation will develop. Make your TA contraction gradually and only up to 25 percent of what you sense would be your maximum effort. If you activate the muscle too strongly or rapidly, you will use its fast twitch fibers. So, go slowly to engage the endurance fibers that will support your abdomen in the long term.

Repeat the above steps several times. Then, when you're sure you're activating the TA, sustain the feeling while you continue breathing through your lower ribs. Start with one full breathing cycle and work up to eight.

If you cannot breathe correctly while holding the contraction, reestablish your starting position to be sure that your lower ribs are free to move before you begin your next attempt. If you allow your lumbar curve to flatten, your outer corset will assume the abdominal work. Because the outer muscles restrict the lower rib cage, they block breathing. Being able to breathe with your lower ribs tells you that you have not engaged the outer corset muscles.

If you are uncomfortable doing this exercise on your hands and knees try bending over from a standing position and leaning your forearms on a table. Allow your knees to be slightly bent. Open your pelvic floor diamond, broaden your shoulders by pressing down on your forearms, relax your belly, breathe, and then follow the instructions for the kneeling version.

Because inner corset practice involves so little effort and produces only internal movement, you may think you're not doing anything. Persist. If you have back pain or a history of back pain, have gone through childbirth, or have had abdominal surgery, you may need three to four months of twice-daily practice to fully develop the TA sensation.

Practice: Activating Your TA Lying Down

Lie down over a folded blanket as you did for supported breathing practice (see fig. 4.2 on page 84). Place a folded towel under your neck and head. Let your shoulders rest back to open your upper chest. The advantage of working in this position is that the blanket supports a neutral position of your lumbar area and opens your lower rib cage for breathing. This makes it harder for you to use your outer corset when you attempt to sense your TA.

Research shows that the TA engages automatically at the end of an exhalation. In this practice, you simply make use of that fact. Rest one hand lightly across your abdomen below your navel. At the end of an exhalation, gradually draw your lower abdomen inward, away from your hand, and upward, toward your back waist. You should sense a gentle hollowing-out feeling within your lower belly. The sensation is of mild internal activity, not of strenuous contraction. Remember, a 25 percent contraction is more than enough.

To check whether the multifidi connections are working, slip one hand between the blanket and your lumbar spine. When you contract your TA, you should not feel pressure down onto your hand, which would indicate that your spine is flattening. Instead, you should feel only a slight swelling or hardening of the lumbar muscles.

Once you feel confident about maintaining the sensation of inner support while you breathe, you can practice it in upright positions. Begin by standing neutrally. Distribute your weight evenly over both feet, release your back triangle, and breathe in three dimensions. If you tend to hold your pelvis in a backward tilt, allow your pubic bone to sink toward your ankles. This should induce a neutral curve in your lumbar spine that, in turn, will lift your rib cage, upper spine, and neck.

If you're aware of having an exaggerated lumbar curve, sometimes called "sway back," you need to produce more length in your lumbar area by elongating your whole spine. Practices in several later chapters will help you develop this. For now, let the crown of your head ascend toward the ceiling. Then, imagine your sacrum sinking heavily toward the floor, without using your buttocks muscles to tuck your tail under.

When you feel that you've achieved a neutral stance, place one hand on your lower belly and the other against your lower back. After an exhalation, slowly pull in and up through your lower belly, drawing your abdomen away from both hands. Sustain your contraction while you continue breathing into your lower ribs.

You can easily practice engaging your TA while waiting for internet help lines, grocery lines, traffic signals, or traffic snarls—any time you have to "hurry up and wait." The practice, because it involves slowing your breathing—thus managing your body's reaction to stress—lets you keep your cool and strengthen your inner corset at the same time.

Practice: A Shortcut to the Inner Corset

Remind yourself about the two fan-shaped ilia that form the sides of your pelvis. Place your thumbs on the sharp points on either side of the front of your pelvis, the anterior superior iliac spines, or ASISs. Then move your fingers back to the dimples on either sides of your sacrum. When the TA is working as it should, it draws these four points together. You can activate your inner corset by visualizing this. Stand neutrally. Imagine your two ASISs moving toward one another at the front of your pelvis and the two dimples drawing together in back. Alternatively, imagine that your two iliac bones are magnetized and are drawing together toward the center of your belly.

If that's all there is to it, you may wonder why we bothered with the other practices. It's important to be very precise about the inner corset sensation because it can so easily be masked by the activity of the outer muscles. This practice serves as a shortcut when you have already learned to distinguish the feeling.

When to Activate Your TA

Walking is an ideal way to challenge and develop your inner corset. You must first be sure that you can clearly perceive the drawing-in action of your TA and then practice sustaining it for longer and longer periods of walking. Stop periodically to recheck the TA sensation. If your outer corset takes over (you will know this because it will become difficult to breathe through your lower ribs), you'll be defeating your purpose. Continue with your lying-down or kneeling practice until your TA becomes stronger.

Another way to develop your TA is to use poor habits as signals to engage it. Do this when you notice yourself leaning on things, for example, the kitchen sink while you're doing dishes. You'll probably find that the work gets done more quickly when your inner corset is engaged. Check your TA whenever you're tired of doing a task or are just plain tired.

Your goal should be to sustain mild tone in your inner corset whenever you're upright. When you're active, the contraction should be 10 to 25 percent of your maximum. Daily practice of the inner corset exercises will make the TA sensation more familiar. The more you feel its benefits to your posture, the more automatic engaging it will become.

Developing central support will make it possible for you to let go of misplaced stabilizing tensions in your shoulders. Because you'll feel more fluidness in your walking and more ease of motion in everything you do, you won't want to ever lose the support of your TA again.

Inner corset support also has an emotional aspect. The muscles surrounding the body's core help us contain energy and emotion—our "gut feelings" and "butterflies." Too much tension in the abdomen can indicate that emotions are being stifled. Flaccid core muscles can shuttle tension to other parts of the body, for instance, engaging jaw or shoulder muscles in "keeping it together." You need core support whenever you feel like giving up on something or are challenged beyond your comfort zone. Attention to your TA can summon unexpected resources for dealing with difficult situations.

Carmen's 10 Percent

Carmen has been juggling her Target job with pre-med courses at city college and workouts at the gym. She tries to watch her diet and spend time with her family, two things that often conflict because her family loves to eat. Sometimes it's just too much. Last week she lost control of her temper and her manager scolded her for snapping at a customer.

Lately, though, she's been practicing what she calls her "bikini squeeze." Her cue to remember it is a tiny twinge in her back. A 10 percent effort is all it takes. The shrinking feeling in her belly interrupts the back pain and makes everything else feel lighter too. Maybe it's all in her head, but she feels less harried by her busy schedule and less apt to "lose it" when a customer is rude. Besides, she's just met a guy. . . .

Coordinating Inner and Outer Corsets

The activity of your inner corset is fundamental to the open stabilization of your posture. However, the inner and outer abdominal muscles do need to work together—the inner muscles for continuous support and the outer ones for strength and movement. The following practice will challenge your inner corset by increasing the load on your spine.

Practice: Flying Table

Assume the table position, as illustrated in fig. 5.4 (p. 100), on a carpeted floor or exercise mat. Engage your TA and then gently press your hands and left shin into the floor as you slowly slide your right foot out behind you until your knee is straight. Sustaining your TA contraction and breathing steadily, lift your right leg until it is in line with your trunk. Keep your kneecap facing down toward the floor. Avoid turning your leg outward when lifting it up.

You may feel yourself leaning into your left hip as you raise your right leg. To avoid this, push firmly down into the carpet with your left shin and the top of your foot as if you were trying to make an imprint in the carpet with your leg. If your ankles are too stiff for your shins to touch the floor, place a folded towel under them and press against that.

To prevent your shoulders from collapsing as you lift your leg, press down with your hands as if to make handprints in the carpet. Keep your elbows straight but not locked. Broaden your chest and collarbones and keep your shoulder blades down along your back. Have your neck in line with your spine and let your eyes gaze at the floor twelve inches in front of you. Once you feel steady extending your leg, practice the following sequence of actions. Do at least three repetitions on each side, at least once a day. Build up to holding each leg lift for six slow breaths. You should do the following:

1. Check your starting position.
2. As you exhale and engage your TA, slowly slide one leg behind you and then lift the leg in line with your trunk.
3. Hold the position for at least one full breathing cycle.
4. Slowly lower the leg to the starting position while sustaining your TA contraction.
5. Repeat with the other side.

When the leg lift is easy, which could require several weeks of daily practice, add the extension of your opposite arm. After you've extended your right leg, slide your left hand forward along the floor and then lift your straight arm up to trunk level. Recheck all the details: continuous lower rib cage breathing, pelvic floor open, lumbar curve steady, TA secure, chest open, and shoulders broad and down. To keep from collapsing into your supporting hip or shoulder, press firmly into the carpet with your supporting shin and hand. Lower your arm and leg in a gradual, controlled manner and repeat with the other side.

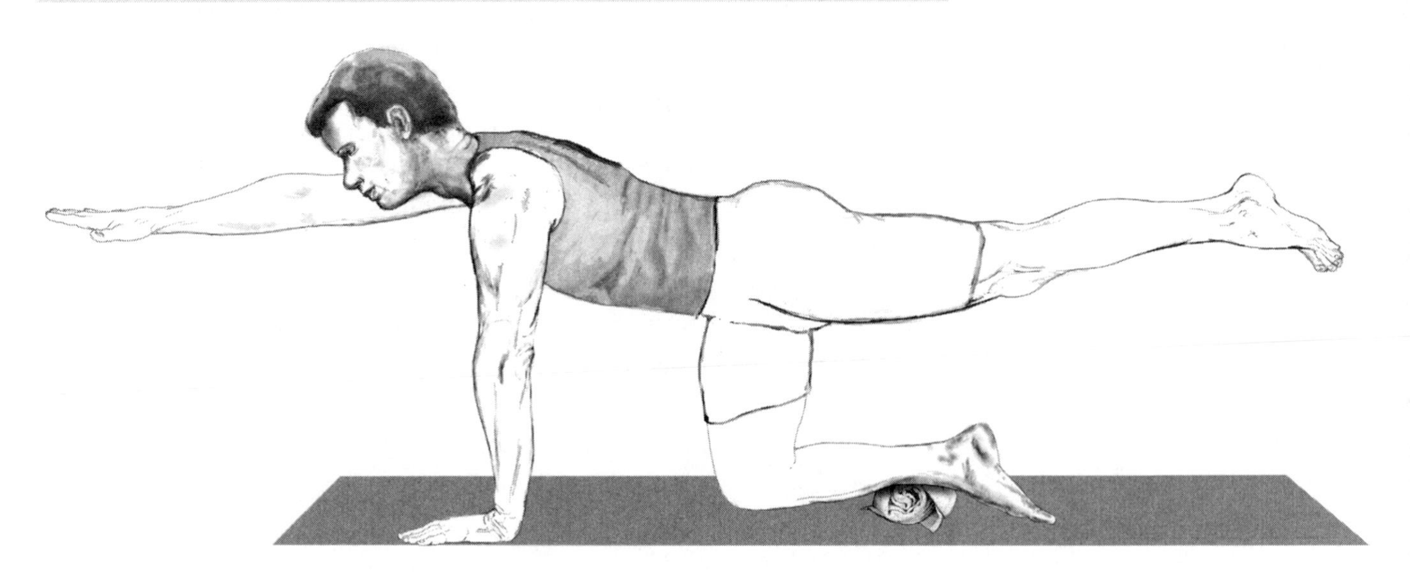

Fig. 5.5. The Flying Table practice. By extending your arm and leg, you challenge your ability to sustain the TA contraction.

When you are confident that you can engage your inner corset, omit the other TA practices in favor of this one. Do three or four careful repetitions daily. This exercise, in addition to challenging your TA, strengthens the postural muscles that are used for healthy walking. As you lift your leg, be aware of activity in your buttock muscles. You're not aiming for "buns of steel," but the sensation of activity in your buttocks is one of the secrets of healthy walking. This is why it's important not to turn your leg outward when you lift it. To do so would train your hips for a Charlie Chaplin walk—not what you want. We will explore walking in detail in chapter 9. For now, notice how your walking feels after you've practiced the Flying Table several times on each side.

Engaging Your Inner Corset During Exercise

If you can maintain core support and steady breathing during the Flying Table practice, you are ready to incorporate healthy core support into your customary exercise program. Because not all fitness instructors know how to help you activate your inner corset, keep the following four rules in mind:

- Feel for your TA sensation before and during any exercise.
- Reconnect with your TA if you notice your abdomen protruding.
- If your pelvis tucks under, reopen your back triangle and/or drop your pubic bone.
- Be sure that your lower rib cage expands in all three dimensions as you breathe.

Your Inner Corset in Daily Life

Body awareness plummets when you're intensely focused on getting a job done. Yet it's when you're not thinking about your body that you need support the most. Train yourself to engage your inner corset first in situations that require extra stability—lifting a five-gallon water bottle, for example, or a heavy suitcase. In such tasks, the outer muscles are working, too, but it is only the inner corset that can prevent your vertebrae from compressing under the load.

Spend a little time redesigning the way you do simple daily tasks and practice the new versions until they become automatic. The next exploration will show you how inner corset support helps with mundane activities such as bending over, straightening up, and lifting heavy objects.

Exploration: Bending Forward and Bending Down

The Bending Over exploration in chapter 3 (p. 65) introduced the action of bending forward by using your hip joints as hinges. Review that motion. Start from the healthy sitting position and then lean forward, widening your back triangle. Let your pubic bone rest down and your tailbone rise slightly. Then repeat, adding abdominal support to the action. Draw your lower belly in and up just before you lean forward. To return to an upright posture, sustain the TA sensation while you push down through your feet for leverage. Repeat with awareness until this feels comfortable and easy.

Many forward bending actions require both folding the hips and curving the upper spine. Try this now: from a seated position, lean forward from your hip hinges until you approach a forty-five-degree angle with your trunk. Then, while sustaining your inner corset support, curve your chest and shoulders forward as if bending to tie your shoes. To return sitting upright, raise your upper spine first and then push down with your feet to reopen your hip angle.

Whenever you combine these two actions, bending the hips should precede moving your chest and shoulders. This is true even when the movement is very small, such as bending forward to take a bite of food. Try it. While seated at a table, incline your trunk forward as if toward your plate. This will probably feel unfamiliar. Most people slouch forward with the upper trunk and shoulders when they eat.

Experiment with bending over from the standing position. Stand at your bathroom sink and bend over to wash your face. If you're like most people, you bend over from the waist. Instead, bend your knees a little, engage your core support, and lean forward from your hips. Then let your shoulders fold forward. Be sure you have not narrowed your sit bones or tucked your tail under. To straighten up, reopen your chest and push down with your feet.

Some movement therapists teach straightening up from the bent position as a "rolling up" action through the lumbar spine. Although this is useful for developing sequential action between individual vertebrae, doing it in daily life, especially without core support, is a lower back problem in the making.

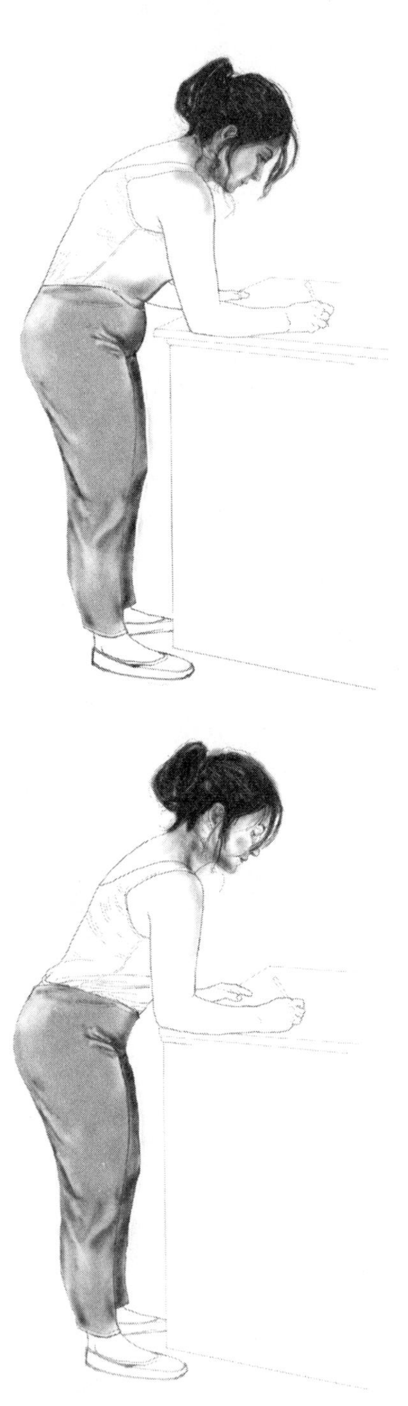

Fig. 5.6. Carmen stopped experiencing back pain when she learned to bend over correctly, as shown in the lower image.

Now explore bending much farther. Simultaneously draw in and up through your TA, bend your knees and fold forward from your hip joints as you reach down to pick up a pencil from the floor. Wait until your trunk is parallel to the floor before curving your upper spine and shoulders. If this style of bending over feels unfamiliar, you will need to attend to it patiently until you have revised your habit.

Whether you bend over to sign your name, make the bed, put on your pants, or feed the cat, the rules for bending and straightening are the same:

- Be sure of inner corset support before you move.
- Bend forward before bending down (folding at the hip hinges before folding above the waist).
- To rise, unfold your upper back and then push down with your feet to straighten your hips.
- Avoid compressing your pelvic floor before, during, or after bending.
- When you bend from a standing position, use your knees as well as your hips.

Your inner corset, with its fascial connections to the deepest spinal muscles, protects your lower back from forces placed on it when you bend and straighten. This protection becomes critical when you lift something heavier than a pencil. Observe yourself the next time you carry a bag of groceries that is too heavy for its flimsy handles. Many people support such a burden by thrusting the pelvis in front of the chest so that the abdomen becomes a shelf to rest the bag on. Because this involves tucking the tail under, it puts the lumbar spine in the worst possible posture for supporting a load.

If you can't lift a heavy object while following the rules for healthy bending, then the burden is simply too heavy for you. In addition to cultivating healthy posture, you need to do some strength-building exercise. For now, make two trips. You'll get an extra workout from the walk.

Pay special attention to your core support when lifting things out of the back seat or trunk of your car. Such actions usually involve twisting in combination with bending and straightening. Combining these movements is when many backs "go out." Carrying a toddler is another risk. A two-year-old child's antics make him very heavy cargo. Not only do you need core support for your back, you also need core containment on an emotional level—to support your patience.

Core Stability, Breathing, and Your Pelvic Floor

Core support fosters healthy breathing and healthy breathing supports the core—a win/win situation. Both depend on the spine's foundation in the pelvis. When we sit or stand with a neutral lumbar curve, the rib cage rises. Then, when we engage the TA, the diaphragm spreads its force outward to expand the lower ribs. Breathing through the lower ribs, in turn, prevents overuse of the outer corset muscles and compression of the trunk.

The right relationship between the pelvic floor, diaphragm, and inner corset can even prevent urinary problems. The slight forward tilt of the pelvis in healthy sitting and standing deflects the diaphragm's pressure away from the bladder. Inner corset support further protects the urogenital organs from the pressure of breathing.

If your TA is weak, you may unconsciously bear down internally instead of drawing in and up. Bearing down creates abdominal pressure that feels like, but isn't, core support. The action presses down on the perineum and makes the belly harden and protrude. It's a common reaction when you're doing something effortful or something outside your usual routine, such as moving a couch or pulling weeds, and not giving any thought to your body. When you're feeling pressed for time, the bearing down sensation can feel as though you are internally putting on the brakes. Maintaining this mild tension can become a chronic stabilizing habit that undermines your breathing, your inner corset tone, and the health of your pelvic organs.

Most people take a big breath to stabilize the trunk when they're about to lift something heavy. It's fine to use the breath to initiate stability, but be sure that you are not also pressing your belly outward and holding your breath as a substitute for TA support. Bearing down and holding your breath when you lift things can cause a hernia, a protrusion of tissue through the abdominal wall near the groin. This injury is more common in men than in women.

Hurrying

Being in a hurry is an all-too-common stimulus for closing your posture. At the beginning of chapter 4, you assessed the way that you hurry in connection with your breathing habits. Now that you're more in tune with healthy breathing and are developing inner core support, there's a good chance you'll be able to hurry without hunching over and compressing your body. Try it. In time you'll notice that you can move just as fast while sustaining healthy posture.

Sensing Yourself in Relation to Others

Through awareness of your pelvic floor, breathing, and abdominal core, you've been revising the way you stabilize your body and changing the way you do things. However, transforming your posture goes beyond learning to move differently. For lasting improvement, you must let your changing posture affect your relationships.

Poor posture derives in part from how we regard ourselves in relation to other people. Noticing how healthy posture makes you feel when you are with others is an essential aspect of establishing your new habits. You're more likely to sustain these new habits when you feel an emotional as well as a physical difference in your posture.

Coughing

The relationship between your diaphragm, pelvic floor, and core support is graphically demonstrated in the act of coughing (or laughing, for that matter). If you cough with your pelvis rolled back, you'll feel a tendency to puff out your belly and bear down into your pelvic floor. If you cough while sitting in a slight forward pelvic tilt, you won't feel the same pressure on your bladder. Excessive pressure into the perineum during forceful exhalations can trigger urinary incontinence. When you sense a cough coming on, engage your perineal muscles to cough "in and up" instead of down into your pelvic floor.

EXPLORATION: POSTURE AS RELATIONSHIP

Recall the Stabilizing Actions exploration (p. 30), in which you imagined yourself walking to greet a person whom you perceived as intimidating. Repeat that experiment now, but first take time to establish inner corset support and healthy breathing. Sense the spaciousness of your pelvic floor and the accompanying lift in your rib cage. You will probably notice that this shifts your body's weight ever so slightly forward over your feet. Then look across the room at your imaginary person. Walk toward him. Notice how it feels to make this journey. Notice how you experience the intimidating person's attention. Then repeat the encounter without good core support. Notice how you feel about the meeting this time.

The effect of this exploration will be stronger if your can corral a friend who is willing to keep a straight face while you walk toward him. Pretend he is a stranger. You may be surprised at what you learn from this simple charade. How we perceive relationships is strongly colored by how we stabilize our bodies.

Nick's Success

For Nick, the main thing was not to tighten his pelvic floor. He realized that he'd been clenching his buttocks for years as a way of managing his back pain. At first, releasing the back triangle felt like a loss of control, but he had to admit that the tiny adjustment made it possible to sit up straight without effort. His back no longer ached after a stint in front of the computer.

Abandoning his sit-up routine made Nick nervous at first. Because his outer abs were so strong, it took him a while to recognize the sensation of inner corset support. Breathing helped. He took long walks in the mountains, exhaling slowly and letting the inner corset hug his lower back. The area around his surgical scars even began to itch. It felt as if his back muscles were waking up.

Walking without tucking his tail under was the biggest challenge.

Opening his pelvic floor shifted his weight forward and made his legs work in a new way. It felt like he was propelling himself forward, whereas before he'd been dragging himself along with his feet.

He also found himself acting with more confidence and self-assertion. His life seemed to be turning around. He rescued two climbers who'd been stranded in the mountains by ugly weather and brought them out without any strain on his back. Shortly after that, his anatomy professor asked him to be a teaching assistant in next semester's class.

In this section, you will have gained experience with the three posture zones responsible for stabilizing your core. In the next section, "Orientation," you will learn how your posture is affected by your relationship to the world around you through your hands, feet, and senses. You will see how excess tension in the outlying regions of your body can undermine your core support. You will also learn more about open stabilization, which involves the capacity to recognize and let go of unnecessary tension in your body's periphery.

Part Three

Orientation

A man's feet should be planted in his country,
but his eyes should survey the world.

George Santayana

6 YOUR HEART'S MESSENGERS

Hands make the world each day.

PABLO NERUDA

Try this short experiment. Find a pen and paper and sit at a table. Lean forward as if to write but grip your pen hard, harder than usual. Notice that the compression doesn't stop in your wrist. You will feel tension traveling up through your arm and shoulder blade and spreading to your neck and jaw. You may feel your collarbones jutting forward and your chest narrowing. There may even be tension in your lower body as you stabilize for the writing task ahead. Perhaps you're narrowing your pelvic floor or even bearing down through your belly.

Chances are that you never grip a pen with that much intensity. But at some time during the day you do hold tightly to something: mouse, steering wheel, phone, shopping cart, or unruly child. Perhaps you've held on to an emotion or an opinion. We tighten our grip whenever we are trying to maintain control. The drive to control our circumstances often results in chronic tension of the hands, arms, and shoulders. Such tension indicates that we are stabilizing ourselves with the parts of our bodies meant for interaction and relatedness.

Hands provide our primary interface with our surroundings. Reaching out to touch things is how infants explore the world. It's how they learn about the space between objects. Successive manipulation of objects gives them a beginning grasp of the concept of time. Scientists now believe that the evolution of the brain is inextricably linked with the evolution of the hand. It is even possible that the sequential thinking necessitated by the manipulation of tools is what stimulated prehistoric humans to create words and language. It may be that our hands hold the essence of our humanity.

Your body's vertical posture is the embodiment of your personal stance. Stabilizing your stance has been the focus of our discussion so far. In this chapter, we will address the social dimension of our bodies as expressed through the shoulders and arms. While a balanced stance supports effective expression, your stance also depends on the capacity of the upper limbs to reach out for things and people and, when necessary, to push them away.

Because your shoulders link your hands to your body's core, we begin our exploration of the hands by studying the shoulders. Unless your shoulders are free to move, impulses from your core can't be clearly or strongly carried to your hands. In the second part of the chapter, you will discover how your touch—gentle, sentient, hasty, or forceful—influences how you stand and move.

Alison's New Home

It's a hot Sunday afternoon, and Alison is surrounded by packing boxes. Exhausted by the move, she's collapsed on the floor of her new living room and lies there absently staring up at the light fixture. "Art deco," she muses. "Art deco! How could I not have noticed that before?" Within minutes she's perched on a stool, scrubbing at the tarnished brass. The fixture hangs from a chain, so she has to hold it still with one hand while she rubs with the other. In no time, her shoulders are burning, but she's too excited to stop. She knows enough about antiques to think that this might be the real thing. She checks for her inner corset, knowing that without it she'd never have been able to carry all those boxes. Breathe, she tells herself. But the pain in her neck and shoulders wins out and, for now, the chandelier keeps its grimy patina.

Exploration: A Tour of Your Shoulders

Intense focus on a task overrides body awareness. You see this when you thread a needle or search the Internet. Your hands become so merged with the task that they seem to be separate from your body. Alison's hands have gotten away from her. As she reaches for the chandelier, her shoulder blades fail to secure her arms to their mooring on her spine. To understand this, we will briefly tour the structures that make up the shoulders.

Your two collarbones and shoulder blades, the *clavicles* and *scapulas,* respectively, form a girdle that encircles the top of your spine and rib cage. At the base of your throat is notch formed by the intersection of your breastbone and your two collarbones. Place your left thumb in this notch and left forefinger right next to it on the "head" of your right clavicle. Now reach your right hand forward, back, up and down, as if you were wielding a hairdryer. Feel how your clavicle adjusts to every motion. What you are experiencing is the fact that your hands and arms are suspended from the top of your chest. The spot you're touching—between the collarbone and breastbone—is the only place where your arms connect bone-on-bone to your trunk. Otherwise, your arms depend on soft tissues to hold them in place.

Now walk the fingers of your left hand out along your right collarbone until they come to a flat surface. This epaulette-like outcropping is the upper and outer corner of your shoulder blade. The clavicle and scapula abut here to form the most easily dislocated joint in the body.

Your scapulas are the two triangle-shaped plates that lie on the back of your upper rib cage, held there by muscle and connective tissue. Just below the scapulas' bony epaulettes are shallow sockets into which your upper arm bones fit.

The mobile construction of the shoulder girdle contrasts markedly to the secure fittings of the pelvic girdle. Your thighbones fit into deeply recessed sockets on your pelvis, and your sacrum fits tightly between the two ilia. The looser design of the shoulders renders your hands and arms free to explore your surroundings and express your feelings. It also gives them room to develop bad habits. Your shoulders are not designed to stabilize your stance. In fact, when your shoulders, arms, or hands are used to hold you together, they sabotage the open posture you've been trying to achieve. The next several explorations will help you evaluate your shoulder tension.

Exploration: Closing Your Shoulders

Recall a morning when you were shivering with cold. Draw your arms close to your sides as if you were trying to keep warm now. Most likely your rib cage will narrow, your pelvic floor tighten, and your breath move into your upper rib cage. Although you don't maintain this degree of tension in daily life, experiencing it reveals how tension in your arms imprisons your core.

Exploration: Shoulder Expression

While maintaining a small amount of "cold morning tension" in your shoulders, reach your arms out as if opening them to an embrace. Chances are that you can neither make the gesture nor feel the feeling. Your heart sits at the intersection of your outstretched arms and your stance. Your arms' horizontal action reflects your relationship to the world outside yourself. Extending your hands out into space symbolizes freedom to express your feelings. This freedom relies on an openly stabilized core, a secure foundation (which we explore in chapter 7), and your shoulder girdle's capacity to deliver the impulse intended by your heart to its messengers, the hands.

Exploration: Leverage

Among the muscles that secure the scapulas to the trunk, the opposite actions of the upper and lower portions of the *trapezius* are the easiest to understand. Standing comfortably, raise your arms forward like a sleepwalker. Do it several times, noticing where you feel sensations of muscle activity. Most people feel it at the top of the shoulders and upper arms. You may also feel your scapulas riding forward with your arms, your breastbone drawing in, and your whole body swaying back onto your heels.

Repeat the arm gesture with the following difference: slide your shoulder blades down along your back toward your waist and then raise your arms again. Notice how this change causes your upper arms to seat securely into the shoulder sockets and lets you lift your arms without disturbing the openness of your chest or leaning your body back. It also makes your arms feel lighter.

In the first version, when it felt like you were hoisting your arms from your neck, you were using the *upper*

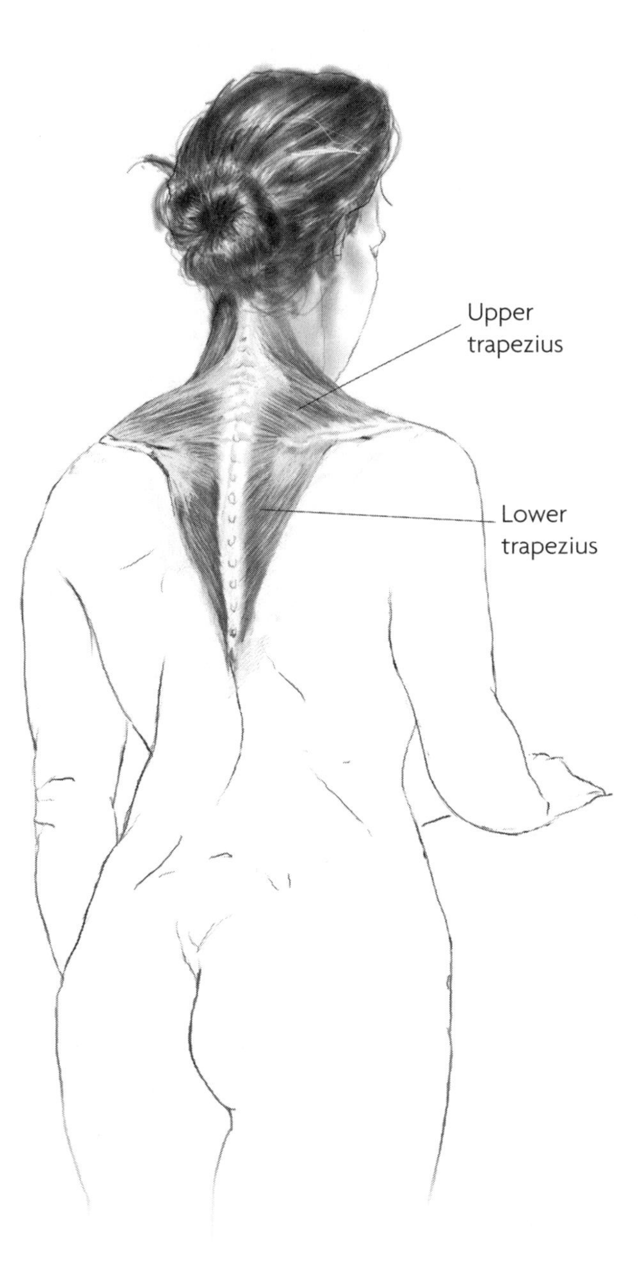

Fig. 6.1. The upper trapezius raises your shoulders toward your neck. The lower trapezius helps secure your scapulas to the middle back, providing a better foundation for movements of your arms.

trapezius. In the second version, your contraction of the *lower trapezius* anchored your scapula to your spine. Stabilizing your shoulders gave your arms better leverage. Most of what we do with our hands involves raising the arms at the shoulder joints, even if only slightly. Whether you're shaking someone's hand, giving them a hug, or blow-drying your hair, the set of your shoulder blades determines how hard your arms must work to maneuver your hands.

Open stabilization of your core is the foundation for healthy use of your shoulders and arms. When your core foundation is secure and your rib cage is open, your shoulders tend to settle back into good alignment. However, because most of us have spent years closing our cores, we habitually carry our scapulas too high on our trunks, making our upper trapezius muscles work far too hard. The next several practices will help you transform this habit.

PRACTICE: SHOULDER BLADE PULSES

Begin by establishing a position of healthy sitting and breathing. Locate the bottom tip of your right scapula (called the *inferior angle*). Reach behind you with your left arm to touch it or look at it in a mirror. Now, using minimal effort of your lower trapezius, draw the tip downward about half an inch and then relax it. Aim your right scapula diagonally down toward your waist. Try this several times. Notice that as your scapula descends, your right clavicle seems to spread and your upper arm bone rotates slightly outward.

The main muscle that draws the scapula down is the lower trapezius. When you relax the pulling-down action, avoid using the upper trapezius to pull the scapula up. Just let it slide up passively. The only muscle that should be active is the lower trapezius. Feel it in the center of your back, just below your shoulder blade. Lightly contract it for less than a second and then let go.

Now the real work begins. Draw your scapula down repetitively with light, pulsing actions. Begin with one pulse per second. In time you can work up to faster pulses as your scapula becomes more coordinated. This is not a strength-building exercise; it's a coordination workout. The problem is not that your lower trapezius is weak but that it's underactive. Lightly activating the muscle in this manner revises the neural circuitry between brain and muscle and creates a new memory of shoulder support.

Repeat the pulses with your left scapula. Feel sensations of activity in the middle of your back, just below your shoulder blade. If your upper trapezius becomes involved, you'll feel activity in your upper shoulder. If so, stop, relax, and begin again. Remember to use inner corset support and to breathe steadily while you pulse your scapulas.

Because the two sides of your lower trapezius differ in their ability to contract and release, they need individual attention. Practice Shoulder Blade Pulses one side at a time. Do them for a few minutes several times daily for three months. Little by little, you will exchange upper shoulder tension for healthy shoulder stability. You can do this at your desk without anyone noticing that you're working out.

You may have noticed that activity in the lower trapezius muscle pushes your rib cage and breasts forward. This correct use of your shoulder girdle helps you lift your rib cage in an open-hearted stance. You can activate your lower trapezius by imagining yourself as the female partner of a couple in ballroom dancing position. The man's hand on your back guiding your steps would be placed across the lower trapezius.

The emphasis on securing the scapulas to the middle of the back does not mean that your scapulas should never slide upward. Releasing the scapulas from the back allows the powerful follow-through of a baseball pitch or tennis serve. You also need that greater range of motion whenever you reach for something on a high shelf or hug someone tall. However, your arms cannot be stable or strong when your scapulas are not secured to your trunk. For the ordinary tasks of daily life, your shoulder blades should rest down along your back rib cage, your clavicles should be broad, and your chest should be open.

Support for the Heart

Even more important for healthy posture than the trapezius muscles are the *serratus anterior* muscles. The serratus muscles are sandwiched between your rib cage and the inside surface of your shoulder blades. They wrap forward through each armpit from the inner edges of your scapulas to midway down the front of your rib cage. In partnership with other muscles that stabilize the scapulas, their action broadens your shoulders by drawing the scapulas flat against your back ribs.

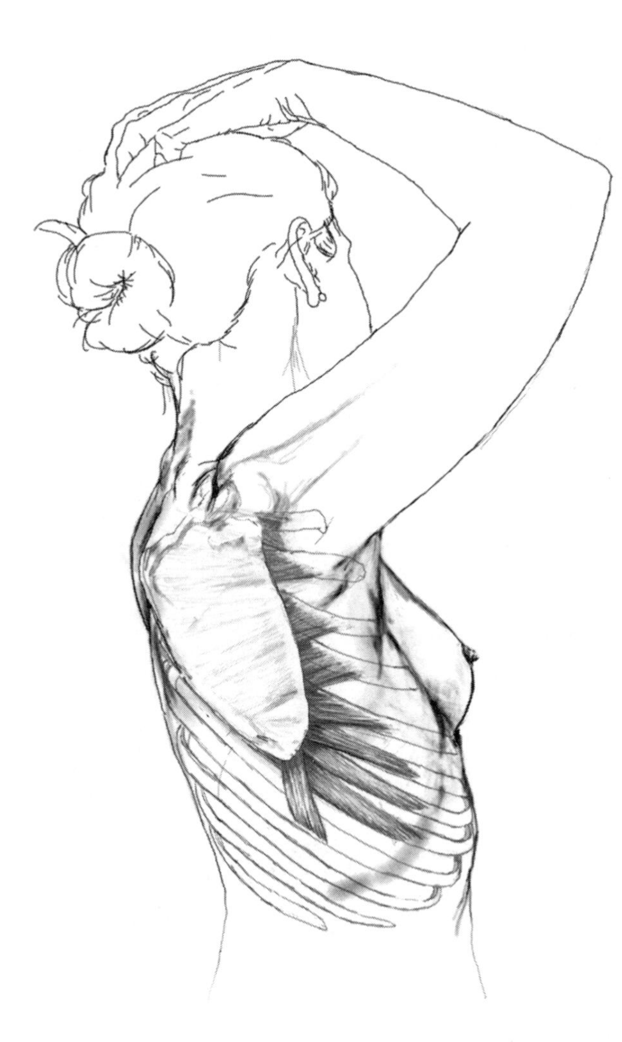

Fig. 6.2. Your serratus anterior muscles give three-dimensional support to your upper body.

Because your serratus anterior muscles wrap from back to front, they give your shoulders three-dimensional support, in contrast to the flat trapezius that secure the scapulas only to the back. The serratus muscles also lie at a deeper fascial layer than other shoulder muscles, closer to your body's core. Further, because of their fascial connections to the upper spine and the abdominal corsets, the serratus anterior muscles form part of two spiraling fascial bands that wrap around your trunk from neck to pelvis.

A fascial pathway runs from the side of the hand near the small finger to the inside edge of the scapula where the serratus anterior attaches. In addition, there is a relationship between the sensory nerves of the hand and the nerves that activate the serratus muscles. Through these connections, tactile awareness in the hands imparts a feeling of adequacy to the shoulder girdle. This, in turn, brings strength and energy to the arms. The following practice will help you sense this.

Practice: Handprints on the Wall

Place a chair facing a wall and sit forward on your sit bones to open your pelvic floor. Engage your inner corset and breathe. Put your hands on the wall so that the heels of your hands are level with your armpits. Sit close enough to the wall to have your elbows slightly bent. Align your middle fingers toward the ceiling and fan the other fingers away from them. Then lightly press your hands into the wall. The goal is to give yourself the impression that your hands and forearms are suspended from the paint. Let your elbows be heavy. If your arms and shoulders do not feel relaxed in this position, adjust the height of your hands or bend your elbows a bit more.

With attention on the effect of your actions in your shoulders, let your skin feel as though it's sinking deeper into the wall, beginning with the pads of your fingers. The action should deepen the sensory awareness of your hands but not involve muscular effort in your arms. Relax any tension that arises in your elbows. When you feel equal pressure through all ten finger pads, gently press with the mounds between your finger joints, and then your palms, until every millimeter of skin on your fingers and palms has equal contact with the paint. The amount of your pressure is slight, no more than an ounce. It can help to imagine that the wall is padded or made of clay.

The movements of your hands are so small that someone watching would probably not notice what you are doing. However, the deepening pressure will begin activating your serratus anterior muscles and produce a subtle shift in the set of your shoulders. Notice any difference in response between your two hands and give extra attention to your less coordinated hand and shoulder.

To further activate the serratus muscles, imagine that your fourth and fifth fingers are growing longer and stretching the skin on the outside edges of your hands. The spreading skin pushes up and out against the wall. Notice how this tiny action stimulates your shoulders. The sensation should travel through your armpits to your shoulder blades, subtly broadening your upper back.

Remain in this orientation for several breathing cycles. Notice that the width in your upper back makes room for your breath to move into your back rib cage without diminishing the openness across your chest. You may also notice a curious sense of ease and freedom in your neck. The support created by the healthy

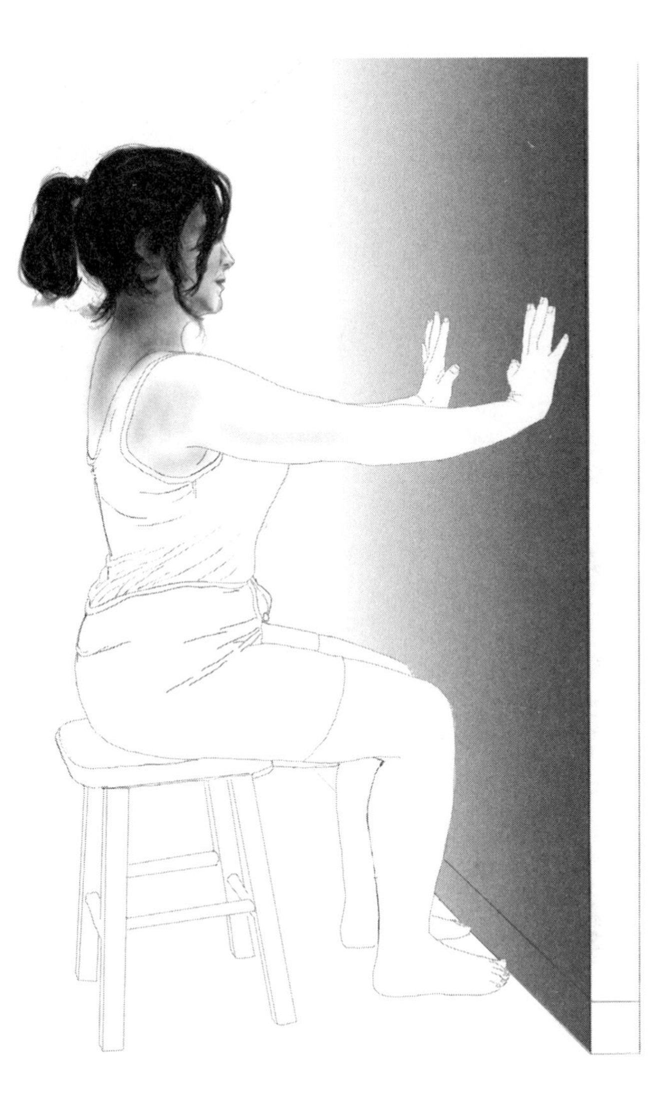

Fig. 6.3. Carmen practices Handprints on the Wall.

orientation of your shoulders provides a foundation for your neck and head.

Sustain the new width in your upper back as you lower your hands from the wall. Stand up and notice how this change affects your stance. Register any subtle shifts in your perception of your surroundings. If there are people nearby, notice how the new feeling in your shoulder girdle affects the way you view them.

Protruding scapulas, sometimes called winged scapulas, are the result of underactive serratus anterior muscles. This postural problem is more prevalent in women than in men. If your shoulder blades protrude, the Handprints on the Wall practice is important because it integrates your shoulders with the way that you use your hands and arms.

The Power of the Small Fingers

Many of us have an unconscious bias toward the thumb side of the hand. Test this out next time you chop a zucchini or polish your car. Notice whether your fourth and fifth fingers are actively engaged in your grasp of a knife handle or polishing cloth. It is common for the small fingers to be underactive. Including them in activities can be surprisingly beneficial to the posture of your whole body.

The bones, muscle, and fascia of the underside of the arm link the fourth and fifth fingers to the shoulder blade and spine. This makes the small fingers important contributors to the power behind any action of the hand. In contrast, the thumb and forefingers connect to the part of the forearm that rotates at the elbow joint. This makes these fingers better suited for manipulation and follow-through. In chapter 7, you will discover a similar division of labor within the anatomy of the foot.

To sense how your different fingers connect to your shoulders and torso, try the following experiment. Place your hands on the steering wheel of your car in the standard "ten and two o'clock" position for driving. Gently squeeze the steering wheel with the emphasis on your small fingers. When you do this, you'll probably feel a subtle sensation of activity underneath your scapulas. For contrast, squeeze the wheel with the emphasis on your thumbs and forefingers. This will produce sensations of activity in your neck and around your collarbones. This experiment is not meant to imply that you should grip your steering wheel tightly when you're driving. Instead, use the "baby's grasp" introduced later in this chapter.

When we hold things in our hands without fully engaging the fourth and fifth fingers, we lose the stabilizing connection between the hands, shoulder blades, and spine. Lacking this connection, we seek stability with the upper trapezius. This leads to the all-too-familiar sensations of neck and upper shoulder tension. It also sabotages the relationship to the abdominal corsets that the serratus muscle can provide.

The next time you polish your car or chop vegetables, engage your small fingers in holding the polishing cloth or knife. Don't overdo it. Simply make your small fingers as actively engaged with the tool as the other three. If you energize your little fingers as you handle everyday objects, you can train your shoulders while you're getting things done. To increase the benefits of those exercises, add tactile awareness of your hands and fingers to the Curling and Arching practice in chapter 2 and to the Flying Table practice in chapter 5.

Practice: Serratus Shortcut

When you've identified the sensation of serratus anterior activity in your shoulders and upper trunk, you can access it readily with this simple exercise. Imagine the skin creases at the backs of your armpits being drawn forward toward the centers of your armpits. Do this when you practice Shoulder Blade Pulses to achieve a three-dimensional result from that exercise. Try it when you're sitting at your desk or driving your car. Do it while putting on your pants or lifting bags of groceries.

Practice: Seated Sphinx

Here's a simple practice to do at your workstation. It's a great refresher for healthy posture when you're in the thick of things. Begin with healthy sitting and healthy breathing. Then lean forward from your hips and spread your forearms, palms, and fingers on your desk. Have the tips of your elbows just off the edge. Allow your upper body to cave in and your shoulders to rise. This will feel as if you're hanging from your shoulder joints, and yes, it's the opposite of healthy posture.

Now press your fingers, palms, and forearms evenly into the desktop as you draw your chest forward. You must release your pelvic floor and let your pubic bone rest down to do this. Use the serratus shortcut. As your shoulder blades flatten down onto your back, you will feel as if your chest is drawn forward through your shoulders. This process links your hands to their support system in your spine.

EXPLORATION: REACHING

Review the Bending Over exploration from chapter 3 (p. 65) in which you practiced bending forward using your hip joints. Now you'll add a reaching gesture to the mix. Pretend you're about to reach across your desk for the stapler. Before you do so, activate your serratus muscles to broaden your upper back. Then reach forward by bending at your hip joints. Allow your arm and scapula to follow through. Unless the stapler is very far away, you won't need to raise your shoulder or close your chest. Notice that when you reach out in this manner, you reach with an open heart as well as with an open hand.

Compare this manner of reaching with a closed version. Sit with your pelvis rolled back and then reach forward for the same object. Because you are now bending from your waist instead of your hips, the stapler seems farther away. To reach it you let go of your shoulder blade, which swings your collarbone forward. This closes your chest and heart area. This is inefficient because you are moving both toward and away from what you want.

Take a moment to appreciate your outlook during the two versions of this simple action. It's just a stapler, but you may notice a subtle difference in how you perceive it. Reaching forward physically is a metaphor for reaching out for what you want in general—for people, for experiences. Imagine that the stapler represents a friendship, a trip to Italy, or a promotion. Compare the two different ways of reaching for what you want. The ability to reach out wholeheartedly contributes lift to your posture.

The ability to freely reach out for things also expands your spatial orientation, a consideration that we will discuss further in chapter 9. When your posture is too closed to reach out wholeheartedly, your awareness of your surroundings—and of your possibilities—tends to be limited.

Carmen's Kitchen Tango

Carmen and her mother are cleaning up after a big family party. A buxom woman, Theresa leans heavily against the sink while scouring a crusty pan. A mountain of dishes is beside her on the counter.

"Move over, Mamacita," says Carmen. "I'll get that done in no time." Twenty minutes later, Carmen's back has begun to ache. She glances at her

reflection in the window above the sink. She might as well be looking at her mom. Her hips are thrust forward to lean on the counter and her shoulders are bunched over the sink. Love for her mom aside, she'd rather not borrow her mother's posture.

She senses the "belly brakes" pushing her abdomen forward. "Bikini squeeze," she mutters to herself, taking a breath and opening her chest. Then she remembers an imaginary dancing partner's hand on her back. She hums a tango. When she does that little armpit trick, her elbow shoots forward like a piston. With her shoulder blades as counterweights to the motion of her arm, the crusty plates come clean more easily.

She invents a mantra: "bikini squeeze and armpit twirl." It slows her down at first, but she likes the light feeling it gives her. A samba might speed things up. She wonders if that cute lab assistant in her anatomy class can dance. . . . Nick, wasn't that his name?

Arm Swing

The Walking Inventory exploration in chapter 1 drew your attention to your usual arm swing. Compare that walking style to what happens now. Find healthy core support, breathe in three dimensions, activate your serratus, and then walk. If you've been able to change the orientation of your shoulders, you'll feel your arms swinging from your back. If you can't feel this yet, you may find the solution in the next practice.

Arm swing is an essential component of walking. The whole body is affected when arm swing is reduced. A study of breast cancer patients showed that 65 percent of the women studied had decreased arm swing on the side of the affected breast. When tested for mobility, the women were found to have no physical restriction in their shoulders. This implied that they had unconsciously suppressed their spatial awareness on the diseased side, which in turn suppressed the swinging of the arm. Loss of motion became more pronounced after mastectomy. For some women, the reduced arm swing led to compensatory hip imbalance and lower back pain.*

Although response to illness can restrict movement anywhere in our bodies, this research points up the potential relationship between shoulder tension and lower back pain. Apart from illness, common causes of shoulder tension are the use of shoulder bags, backpacks, and cell phones. For the health of your spine and shoulders, take heavy items out of your purse or backpack and, whenever possible, walk with your arms unencumbered by

Dowager's Hump

Some women will find that healthy posture projects their breasts forward more than is emotionally comfortable. Cultural confusion about women's roles has led to a habit of holding the breastbone down as a way of minimizing or protecting the breasts. This pattern drags the collarbones down, which in turn pulls the head and neck forward. The resulting strain on the base of the neck can cause an unattractive buildup of connective tissue there. In later life such exaggerated curvature of the upper spine can become extreme and can lead to a condition known as dowager's hump. Allowing your chest and breasts to come forward can help prevent this from happening.

*Hubert Godard et al., "Motion ed E-Motion in Oncologia," in *Psiconcologia*, edited by D. Amadori et al. (Milan: Masson, 2001), 875–81.

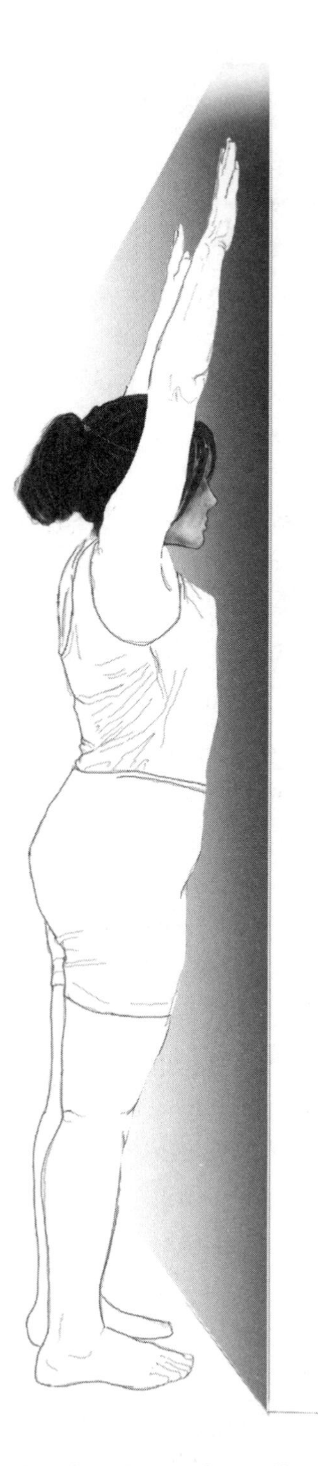

Fig. 6.4. Position for Wall Traction practice.

phones and bags. Add the feeling of freely swinging scapulas and arms to your growing repertoire of healthy posture sensations. The next practice will give your shoulders more freedom to swing.

Practice: Wall Traction

This practice will release tension in your shoulders and rib cage and help to decompress your spine. Do it in small doses if your shoulders are tight. Gradually work up to the full stretch. Stand with your toes about three inches from a wall. Have your feet hip-distance apart. Release your pelvic floor. Rest your lower breastbone on the wall, lifting your breasts if necessary. Rest your forehead on the wall. (It may scrunch your nose a bit.) Spread your hands on the wall beside your ears with your elbows hanging down. Breathe steadily through your lower ribs.

Inch your hands up the wall and over your head. Straighten your elbows as much as is comfortable while keeping your forearms in contact with the wall. When your hands are as far up as they can comfortably reach, press the skin of your palms and fingers to the wall. Draw the backs of your armpits forward. Rest in the stretch for three slow, moderate breaths.

Release your arms from the wall gradually. Then step back and feel what the stretch has done for your body. You will probably feel taller and more open through the trunk. This is a taste of the healthy posture you are gradually redeeming. The more you let yourself sense it, the more familiar and integrated it becomes. Consciously sustain the open feeling as you walk around. Notice how the stretch may have affected your arm swing.

Practice Wall Traction twice a day or whenever you sense your shoulders tensing and your core closing. Work up to eight slow breaths to give yourself a full minute in the stretch.

Carmen's Back Bend

Carmen doesn't know how to explain her recent feat. She did a back bend! It's a crazy thing to get so excited about, but she'd been the only person in the yoga class who couldn't do that pose, even after a whole year. Today it happened like magic, as if she'd always been able to do it.

What Carmen doesn't realize it that by opening her pelvic floor and allowing her breasts to come forward, she released tension in her trunk that kept her spine from arching. What's thrilling is not that she can do this yoga pose but that she can now fully inhabit her womanly body.

REPETITIVE MOTION INJURIES

When you use a hammer, fishing rod, or comb, your tool becomes a temporary extension of your body. Highly developed integration of his body with his golf clubs has made a champion of Tiger Woods. Integration of his body and his cello bow has made a virtuoso of Yo-Yo Ma. However, intense focus on manipulating a tool, especially when the rest of your body is still, can so overwhelm your awareness that your body becomes an extension of the tool rather than vice versa. When your hand on the mouse becomes part of the computer, it is easy to lose connection between your heart and hand—between how you feel and what you're doing. Closed stabilization and shoulder tension then replace open posture.

Hand and arm injuries disable hundreds of thousands of Americans every year and cost the country billions of dollars in compensation, lost wages, and decreased production. In the case of computer use, repetitive motion injuries are probably caused less by motion and more by rigidity of the hand and arm between moves. Frequently, the mouse is gripped as if one's life depended on the outcome of the next click. Just as when you tightly grasped your pen at the beginning of this chapter, your grip on a mouse sends strain through the muscles and fascia of your arm all the way to your neck. There it colludes with the tension created by your eyes being glued to a monitor. Even those who use trackballs tense their arms and shoulders in readiness to move and click.

If you have been plagued by hand pain caused by computer use or other repetitive motion, it will be helpful for you to understand the anatomy involved. The nerves to your hands weave through the scalene muscles on the side of your neck (see chapter 1) and pass under your clavicles and down your arms. The area between the clavicles and rib cage is called the *thoracic outlet.* When the clavicles are drawn forward by closed posture, this passageway for the nerves narrows. If closed posture of the shoulder girdle becomes habitual, fascial adhesions can entrap the nerves. Overuse of the scalenes for upper chest breathing can also restrict the thoracic outlet. Therefore, sometimes hand pain is caused by an anatomical problem higher up in the body.

Precision Activities

If your occupation involves using your hands with delicacy or precision—surgery, dentistry, or hairstyling come to mind—then you will need to practice the new coordination of your shoulders and hands while you do your work. Bring some of your tools home and revise your way of using them on something that won't threaten you with a lawsuit.

And sometimes hand pain is due to a problem in the hand itself. The carpal bones are eight tiny bones in the heel of each hand. Two of these bones have bumps that make those bones stick up higher than the others to form the infamous carpal tunnel. You can feel the bumps if you press on the heel of your hand just past your wrist at the bases of your thumb and little finger. The nerves and the blood vessels that supply your fingers run through the narrow crevice between these bones. The tendons of the many forearm muscles that are used to move your wrist and hand also pass through this tunnel. Carpal tunnel syndrome is a collection of painful symptoms that result when tension in the forearm compresses the tunnel and diminishes the blood supply to the nerves of the hand. By restoring healthy posture, you can reduce or eliminate many types of arm and hand pain.

Loss of body consciousness is a hidden downside of the convenience and power of the electronic age. To keep your hands free of pain and to maintain the health of your posture, it is crucial to take breaks to move your body when doing computer work. Any of the practices in this chapter will help. Movement interrupts the hypnotic quality of the electronic workplace and is a healthier way to restore yourself than snacking or drinking caffeine.

Laptops

By now you've learned enough about healthy posture to suspect that constant use of a laptop computer is not good for your posture. It's hard to sit in a healthy way with a laptop on your lap and next to impossible for your shoulders to be broad. Whenever possible, connect your laptop to a separate keyboard and position the monitor high enough for your core to be open and your head erect.

Practice: First Aid for Your "Mouse Arm"

This practice stretches the fascial pathway through which the nerves to your hands run. Stand sideways to a wall and about two feet away from it. Place your right hand on the wall with the heel of your hand at the level of your armpit and your elbow slightly bent. Spread your fingers so that every possible millimeter of skin on your palm and fingers touches the wall. Check your stance. Release your pelvic floor, engage your inner corset, draw the back edges of your armpits forward, and breathe slowly and moderately. Adjust your stance so that your elbow points directly down at the floor. In this position, you should feel a breadth across your clavicles. You may also begin to feel a burning sensation through your arm as the stretch releases fascial adhesions that have been trapping the nerves. Breathe! Tolerate a moderate degree of the burning sensation while holding the stretch for at least three slow breaths. Keep your fingers flat against the wall. If you are able to straighten your elbow without raising your scapula, do so. However, keeping your scapula down is more important than straightening your elbow. If your shoulder is quite restricted, you won't need to straighten your elbow to feel the stretch.

When you release your hand from the wall, pause to notice the after effect. The arm you stretched will probably seem longer than the other one. If you experience chronic hand or wrist pain, practice this stretch several times each day during breaks in your work. Work up to sustaining it for eight slow breaths. Be sure to stretch both arms to even out your shoulders.

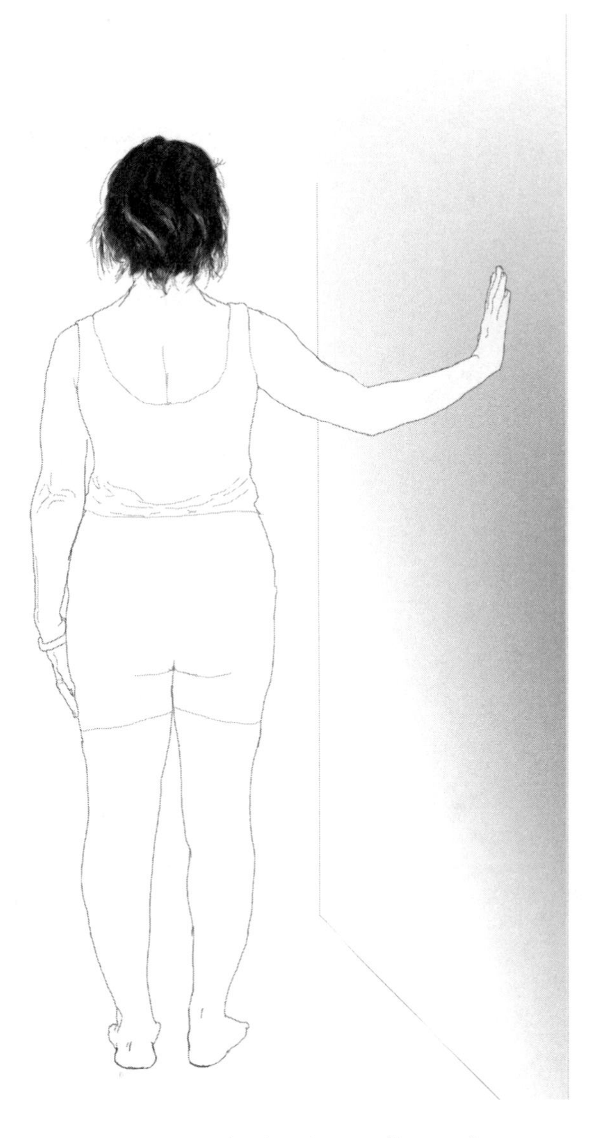

Fig. 6.5. This hand-to-wall stretch can help prevent carpal tunnel or thoracic outlet problems.

Skintelligence

Up to now, this chapter has addressed shoulder support for using your hands. The next section shows you how the way you touch things influences your posture and body use. Tension in your hands communicates throughout your body, confusing your negotiation with gravity and distorting your posture. When you grip things tightly, you are using your hands for stabilization and blocking their expressive and information-gathering gifts.

Because skin and brain derive from the same type of embryonic tissue, it's reasonable to consider your skin as an extension of your brain. I've coined the term "skintelligence" to describe this connection. Your sense of touch—your skin's intelligence—affects the coordination of your whole body.

Certain areas of skin are more sensitive than others. You can feel this for yourself with an experiment. Lightly brush the skin of your upper arm with your fingertips. When you do the same light strokes across your palm, the sensation will be more exquisite. The soles of the feet are also very sensitive. Animal studies show a connection between hairless footpads and reflexive control of movement.* Reflexive coordination is perfectly illustrated by the graceful power of a tiger. It also is what makes elite athletes and actors so extraordinary. They have learned to use their body's skintelligence, and so can you.

*D. Ferrington and Mark Rowe, "Cutaneous Mechanoreceptors and the Central Processing of Their Signals: Implications for Proprioceptive Coding," in *Proprioception, Posture and Emotion,* edited by David Garlick. (Kensington, N.S.W., Australia: University of New South Wales, 1982), 56–69.

To appreciate the link between tactile sensation and coordination, we need first to look briefly at how movement is organized by the nervous system. Muscles are controlled by the interaction of three parts of the brain—the primitive *brain stem,* the ancient *limbic* system, and the more recently developed *cerebral cortex.* Whether you are jerking your hand from a hot stove or snuggling up to a lover, incoming sensations are matched with movement responses. Your primitive brain stem, the so-called reptilian brain, organizes automatic motions such as digestion and heartbeat, emergency acts such as coughing, and reflexes such as a baby turning toward the sound of her mother's voice. The brain stem also monitors learned activities such as walking, bicycle riding, or piano playing after these actions are mastered. The limbic, or mammalian brain, monitors the tactile, kinesthetic, and emotional feel of movement. Movement is most refined and powerful when it is coordinated by these primitive centers.

The sensory-motor part of the cerebral cortex is involved with all movement, but it is especially important when we attempt movements that we have never done before. In the cortical brain, movement is more abstract, more "mental." To know the difference, you need only compare your attempt to master a new dance step, which involves your cerebral cortex, to the grace of your teacher, whose reptilian brain has already integrated the moves.

The organization of movement within the brain is the physiological basis for the emphasis throughout *The New Rules of Posture* on taking time after experiential practice to notice any changed perceptions or mood shifts that may result. You cannot change your habits by commanding your posture with your cortical brain. Instead, you must activate your *subcortical* centers, i.e. the reptilian and mammalian centers, through sensations, perceptions, and emotions.

One of the most effective ways to activate your reptilian brain is to make use of the sensors in your skin. The sense of touch accesses deeper integration within our nervous system than does our muscle sense. Also, because our primitive brain doesn't distinguish between real or imagined events, we can even evoke new coordination by imagining tactile sensations.

The following exploration introduces you to the concept that we receive information about our surroundings through our hands. Touch is a two-way street. Whenever we handle an object, we are also being touched by it. By being unconscious of this two-way exchange, we limit our perceptions as well as our potential for mental, emotional, and spiritual growth.

Exploration: Sacred Touch, Living Touch

Choose a simple, familiar household task such as washing dishes. As you perform the activity, let your hands be attentive to the tactile sensations involved. Feel the weight of each object in your hands. Feel its roundness, flatness, or sharpness. Feel the texture of the sponge, the temperature of the water, and the tickle of soap bubbles. Notice the lightness of your hands after you set something down. Handle the dishes as if you were touching sacred objects or delicate living creatures. Do this for five minutes before reading further.

You probably found that paying attention to the sensory dimension of your activity changed the way your movements were coordinated. Compared with your usual way of doing the task, your shoulders were more relaxed, your breathing was steadier, and you may even have felt your inner corset engaging without being summoned. Although you were moving slowly, your actions were direct and efficient. You got the job done without closing your body. With practice you will be able to sustain that grace while moving at a quicker pace.

A Baby's Grasp

When you hold out a finger for an infant to grasp, the delicate fingers seem superglued around your own. The baby's touch is light, warm, and surprisingly strong. Because a baby's grasp is reflexive, you might even have to pry the tiny fingers away. An elite athlete's grasp of a club or racket has the instinctive skintelligence of an infant. A fully sentient touch allows for precise control, whereas a tight grip actually destroys finesse.

Heavy-handedness evokes resistance. Practitioners of the Japanese martial art form, aikido, use this principle to control their opponents. An opponent instinctively complies with the fighter's gentle grasp, almost as if he were eager to be thrown down.

Most of us manipulate the objects around us without much consciousness. Although we are handling things, we don't really feel what we are touching. Thus, our skintelligence quotient is low. The following practice will help you experience the intelligence of your skin.

Driving

Refer to the box about sitting in car seats in chapter 3 (p. 68) and add what you now know about using your shoulder girdle. Then examine the way your hands contact the steering wheel. When you engage your skintelligence in grasping the wheel, you will sense the road through your hands. This helps keep you alert and connected to the activity of driving. If you grip the wheel tightly, you create unnecessary tension in your shoulders, and are more apt to become dissociated from the activity of driving. If you find yourself daydreaming or getting impatient, shift some attention to your hands and let their skintelligence bring you into the present moment.

PRACTICE: TWO-WAY TOUCHING

Try any household task in the following way. When you grasp your tool, let your hands take in the sensations of the object you are holding. Be touched by what you are touching.

Vacuuming, a task many people dislike, is ideal for this practice. What a chore it is—dragging the clumsy unit out of the closet, untangling the chord, bumping into furniture, and maneuvering the wand underneath the bed. It may sound strange to vacuum with your skin instead of with your muscles, but give it a try. As you set up your machine, let your hands receive tactile impressions at the same time as they move the machine. Let your palm and fingers be touched by the vacuum cleaner. As you grasp the handle, imagine that it is superglued to your skin.

To feel what you are touching, you instinctively loosen your grip. By loosening your grip, you free your arms and shoulders to handle things differently. You might notice that the equipment feels less cumbersome than usual. That is because your tactile sensations ignite the movement centers in your brain stem to organize your coordination and overcome the resistance of your attitude.

Try this trick in other contexts. From folding laundry to shooting hoops, your coordination improves whenever you let your skin help do the work.

Alison's Rules

Alison checks off the chores to be done around her new home. She's discovered that when a job is hard she tucks her tail under, bears down in her belly and lifts her shoulders. It happens over and over. She's made up four rules for healthier body use:

- *Untuck tail, find inner corset, and breathe*
- *Rest shoulder blades on back*
- *Bend over with hips and knees*
- *Feel what I'm touching*

The rules help her constantly but especially whenever she lifts something. Her arms are not very strong, so the rules help her use her body in a way that lets her accomplish more with less effort and less stress.

EXPLORATION: LIFTING SOMETHING HEAVY

Practice with an empty suitcase or other large object. Use Alison's rules as you bend over for the object. Then add the following points:

- Just before lifting, refresh your inner corset.
- Lift by straightening your knees.
- Keep the object close to the center of your body.
- Avoid twisting your trunk.
- Breathe.

These rules apply to lifting anything heavy. Avoid bending and lifting first thing in the morning. Studies show that your lumbar disks are more vulnerable to injury at that time. If lifting something causes you to lose the features of open stabilization, your arms and shoulders may be too weak for the task at hand. Instead of stressing yourself and closing your posture, ask for help. Later, add arm-strengthening exercise to your fitness routine.

Progress

Nick sits in a traffic jam, drumming his fingers on the steering wheel. He's going to be late for the physiology lab he's supposed to be assisting. He can picture the whole class scrutinizing him when he finally makes it in. Especially that girl at the front table. "Carmen. Hmm. . . . C'mon, man, pretty women are trouble," he thinks, "and besides, she's way too young."

He's about to hurl some nasty thoughts at a car that cut in front of him, but just then a twinge in his back makes him shift in his seat. The small movement reminds him to sense his TA. Perhaps the abdominal sensation only distracted him from his irritation, but it seemed to help him contain it. In any case, his hands relax, his breathing slows, his shoulders settle, and his mood gets considerably lighter. Maybe she'd go out for coffee with him sometime. . . .

Alison, too, is making progress. She had her first epiphany in Home Depot, where she'd gone for shelving and a shower nozzle. She was cursing as she struggled to turn the unwieldy cart into the plumbing aisle. At that moment she happened to think about skintelligence, and immediately the cart stopped being an adversary. It was amazing. She's noticed too, that the tingling in her fingers that used to wake her up at night has stopped. She's given up on the chandelier, though. Within minutes of standing on the stool, her neck and shoulders burn. She must be missing something, she thinks. She will find out what that is in chapter 7.

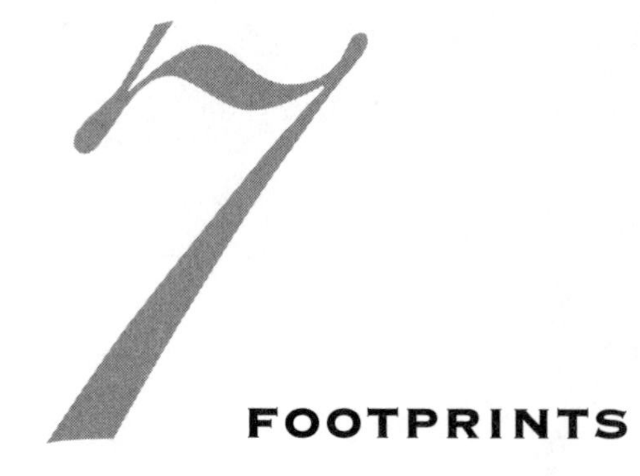

7 FOOTPRINTS

Think of the
magic of that foot,
comparatively small,
upon which your
whole weight rests.
It is a miracle. . . .

Martha Graham

When her children were in their teens, Theresa worked in a factory to supplement the family income. Retired now, she spends most days looking after Rico, her little grandson. He's a handful, that child. It hurts her knees to pick him up, and by the time they get home from the park, she can barely walk. Maybe ten years standing on a concrete floor wasn't so good for her body. Well, her kids are in college; that was always the important thing.

Carmen, her youngest, who is going to be a nurse, has been reading a book that teaches you to improve your posture and, with the enthusiasm of the young, thinks the exercises can help her mom as well. Theresa humors her. After all, what can it hurt to spend time with your beautiful daughter?

They practice opening up the diamond in your pants. Theresa thinks of it as sticking out her bottom, though Carmen says that it's not the same. Then they practice holding the stomach in a special way. Carmen calls it "squeezing your bikini." She tells Theresa to do it whenever she catches herself leaning on the kitchen sink or while she watches TV.

It's been a month now, and the funny thing is, Theresa seems to feel more energetic. There's something else that's hard to name. It's as though the pride in her children that she feels in her mind now shows in her body.

She can walk a little farther every day. Climbing stairs, though, still makes her knees burn.

THE FEET: OUR HUMBLE FOUNDATION

Most people would agree that one of life's pleasures is a luxurious foot rub. By the same token, few things are more draining of good spirits than sore feet. We regard our feet with conflicting attitudes. "Oh, my aching dogs," we say and yet we squander our lunch money to decorate them.

Confusion about feet may have prehistoric origins. Human feet have pheromone-producing glands similar to those in our armpits and genitals. Perhaps, many millennia ago, primitive humans marked their trails with mating signals through foot odor. Cultural and religious taboos about feet may have arisen to curtail sexual promiscuity. Regardless of your own attitude toward your feet, your use of them is as crucial to postural health as steady breathing, core containment, or pelvic mobility.

An engineering maxim concisely states why our feet are so important: "As goes the foundation, so goes the building." Unlike a building, though, our bodies move. Our bodies' foundation must adapt to the uneven surfaces beneath our feet as well as to the motion of the rest of the body above. It must also sustain the repetitive shocks of walking and the sudden impacts of athletics or work. On an average day, our feet absorb up to three million pounds of pressure. When our feet fail at these responsibilities, our whole body suffers. Many therapists consider foot imbalance to be a major cause of low back pain and the source of problems as far away as shoulders, neck, and jaw.*

To dispel any doubt about how profoundly your feet affect your posture, try the following experiment. Walk as if you were going barefoot across an ice-cold floor. Notice how your whole body lifts to help your feet minimize contact with the ground. You do everything you can to resist gravity. Your stride shortens, pelvic floor tucks, shoulders rise, and breathing pauses. Now, still holding extra tension in your feet, pantomime your tennis serve or do some salsa steps. Notice that no joint in your body retains its usual freedom, nor can you feel much pleasure or confidence in your performance.

Your feet, the foundation for your physical stance, also influence your psychological footing. How assuredly you stand on your "own two feet" in expressing your needs and opinions and in fulfilling your responsibilities definitely has a physical base. Many people, like Mika, the neighbor in chapter 1, unconsciously avoid touching the ground, just as you did with the cold floor. Habitual use of the feet in this way turns the legs into stilts. In contrast, other people drag their heels, slogging forward as if their soles were magnetized to the ground.

*Brian A. Rothbart, "Medial Column Foot Systems: An Innovative Tool for Improving Posture," *Journal of Bodywork and Movement Therapies* 6 (2002): 37–46.

The Feet and Health

For more than two millennia, practitioners of Chinese medicine have been treating points on the feet to affect the health of internal organs. A more recent Western healing tradition called reflexology also correlates the organs with specific regions of the feet. Ida Rolf, the founder of Structural Integration, proposed that when feet are properly aligned the reflex points are automatically stimulated by walking.

Tension in the feet, no matter what the cause, restricts their natural movement. This blocks bioelectrical impulses that travel through fascial pathways between the feet and organs. Movement of the feet and legs helps pump lymph and blood to the heart, so anything that restricts movement of the feet also affects circulation. All of this indicates how profoundly the health of the feet affects health in general.

In this chapter, we will explore various ways in which our feet are the foundation of our being. First, we will examine the anatomical features that let us transfer body weight through our feet in walking. We will also work on the alignment of the feet with the knees, hips, and spine. Toward the end of the chapter, we will explore the feet as organs of perception that root, balance, and adapt us to the ground.

Exploration: Self-assessment of Your Feet

Stand in bare feet and pay attention to the pressure of your body's weight against the floor. Stand upright and gaze forward, not down at the ground. Do you feel more pressure on your heels or on the front of your feet? Do you bear more weight to the outer edges of your feet or more to the inside edges? Does one foot feel deeper set into the floor, as if it is bearing more weight?

Now observe yourself while walking. Where does your heel meet the ground: squarely in the center or to the outer or inner heel edge? Are both heels the same?

Consider the middle region of your foot, commonly called the arch. Are you aware of sensation there as you walk?

Do you push off from your toes with a sense that they actively participate in your stride, or do you passively roll over them or scrunch them when you walk? Do you feel the most pressure on the ball of your big toe or can you feel other toes working as well?

Foot Functions

Each part of the foot has a distinct function within each step. The heel is your first contact with the ground. Your heel's touch orients you and tells you where you are. The arch, or midfoot, is responsible for your foot's resilience and adaptability. It is engineered with the precision of a suspension bridge. Many people have high, rigid arches, while other people's arches are nearly flat. The forefoot—from the balls of the foot through the toes—is where your foot finds power. The toes' push-off from the ground completes the action of hip, knee, and ankle to propel your body forward.

If you are like most people, you have little awareness of your midfoot when you walk. Rigidity and collapse in this region are the primary causes of foot problems and compensatory imbalances elsewhere in your body. Poor articulation of the bones in the midfoot prevents smooth transfer of your body's weight from heel to toe. This limits shock absorption and relays the impact of the footfall through muscle, bone, and fascia into the lower spine. To the degree that the upper body braces to withstand this impact, the whole body loses articulation and resilience.

Instead of pushing off from the toes, many people thrust the heel forward and pull the body up to meet it. This style of walking repeatedly displaces the feet ahead of the body and overworks muscles in the hip and thigh. It also engages the toes in gripping the ground and pulling the body forward. This pattern partly explains why so many people have misshaped toes.

Lacking push-off from the toes, some people substitute the knees for this function. By locking the knees shortly after the heel contacts the ground, they use the knees as a fixed point from which to vault the trunk forward. The knee is a relatively simple hinge joint and is thus a poor substitute for the spring-like articulation of the foot. Knee problems that are not caused by injury are often attributable to such repetitive misuse. Rehabilitating the feet often alleviates knee problems.

Anatomy: Stance Foot and Walking Foot

One-quarter of the bones in your body are in your feet. Each foot has twenty-six bones, thirty-two joints, fifty-six ligaments, and thirty-eight muscles. The foundation of your body is clearly a structure designed for very complex movement.

The fluid lining of the joints between the ten bones of the midfoot allows these bones to glide upon one another, somewhat like marbles in a sack. This gliding is what allows your foot to adapt to changing pressures and surfaces. If the midfoot is either overly mobile or extremely rigid, it cannot act like a shock absorber. Unexpected footing will then stress the ankle, a joint that functions like a hinge and is unable to twist. A sprained ankle is often the fault of an unadaptable midfoot.

The bones of the foot form a system of three arches. These include the familiar inside arch that runs from the bottom of the ankle through the first three toes. There is also an outside arch that extends from the heel to the fourth and fifth toes. Finally, a third arch runs horizontally across the ball of the foot. When all three arches are supple, the foot functions as a spring. Upon impact with the ground, the spring absorbs the energy of each step and circulates it back up through the fascial system to contribute to the body's forward momentum.

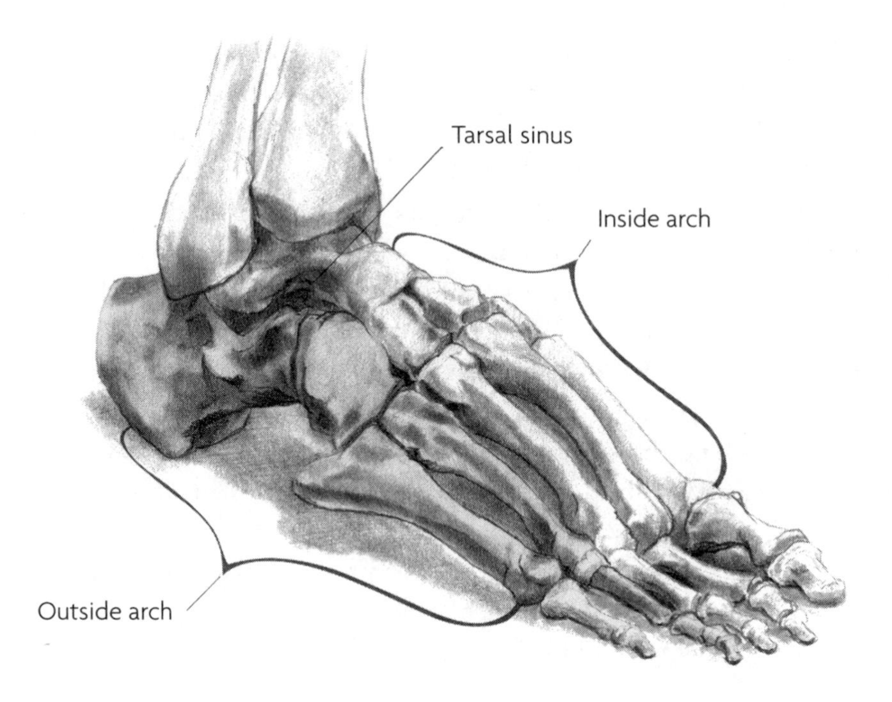

Fig. 7.1. Balance between the outside and inside arches of the foot is the foundation for secure stance and graceful walking.

The outside arch is sometimes called the stance foot because it is responsible for your initial contact with the ground. The inside arch is called the walking foot because its function is to propel your weight forward. The bones that compose the walking foot literally rest on the bones of the stance foot. This design underlies the relationship between stance and movement. That is, how gracefully you walk depends on how securely you stand. Using your feet in accordance with their design minimizes the amount of effort it takes to walk and move.

Exploration: Your Foot's Dimple

While sitting on a chair, bend down and locate a small indentation at the top of your foot. You'll find it just in front of your outside ankle bone (the *lateral malleolus*) and in line with your fourth toe. Surprisingly, this spot (the *tarsal sinus*) marks the front of your heel bone. Most of us conceive of the heel as something on the bottom and back of the foot, a location for calluses. The heel actually makes up the rear third of your foot, a fact that will become important as we go on. While holding a finger in the sinus, cup your other palm under your heel to feel how big it really is.

Scoliosis Footprints

Stand with one foot rolled inward and the other rolled outward. Notice how your pelvis and trunk twist to accommodate to this faulty foundation. This demonstrates how misuse of the feet contributes to rotations in the spine. Such a stance is common with people who have the curvature of the spine called *scoliosis*.

If, during the walking assessment earlier, you noticed a stronger heel strike on one foot, recheck your impression of your footprints when you're standing still. Notice whether you bear more weight on the front of one foot and the heel of the other or whether you stand to the inside of one foot and the outside of the other. If your footprints are uneven, chances are that you have some curvature in your spine. The imbalance in your feet may be compensating for the spinal rotation or vice versa. A strong pattern of this nature, especially if you also experience back pain, can indicate that you need integrative bodywork as well as self-help. Spinal distortions are frequently improved by Structural Integration therapy that includes rebalancing of the feet.

With your foot on the floor and still holding a finger in the sinus, roll your foot to its outer edge. This motion is called *supination*. Notice that it makes the dimple disappear. Roll your foot to the inside and the dimple becomes deeper. This motion is called *pronation*.

In walking, your foot's natural action includes a very slight pronation as it moves from initial contact to push-off. That motion should begin near your tarsal sinus. If your arches are stiff, the rotation takes place farther forward, closer to your toes. This puts excessive pressure on the ball of the big toe.

The tarsal sinus is the functional center of the foot. Across it play the interactions between supination and pronation and movement of the rear foot and forefoot as we stand and walk.

Many people both stand and walk on the walking foot, which means that they stabilize themselves on the part of the foot that is engineered for movement. This leads to overuse and collapse of the inner arch. This pattern, called over pronation or flat foot reduces shock absorption and makes you seek stability elsewhere in your body. It can contribute to bunions, shin splints, pain in the knees or lower back, and tension in the shoulders, neck, or even the jaw.

The following two experiments will help you sense the body-wide ramifications of pronation and supination. Stand with your feet rolled inward onto your inside arches. Most of you will feel a generalized downward tendency in the body and a corresponding poor sense of stability. Take a few steps and notice how you compensate for this poor foundation when you walk. Feel what happens to your pelvic floor, belly, shoulders, and neck when your feet are pronated like this.

Now, stand on the outside edges of your feet, a supinated position. Feel how your upper body reacts. Notice what happens when you walk with your feet like this. People whose midfoot bones form a high, rigid arch walk on the stance foot. This habit reduces the foot's resiliency and usually results in a stiff, side-to-side sway. Supinated feet are often a compensation for pronation, either through the body's instinctive search for stability or as a result of corrective shoes prescribed in childhood.

Foot Practice

The tendons of several calf muscles wrap under your foot to form a stirrup that supports your arches. The tendons intersect beneath the tarsal sinus, where the foot adapts from stance to push-off. If a foot is fixed in either pronation or supination, the tendons adhere to neighboring fascial layers and prevent the natural rotation of the foot.

You've already done one exercise that can help release tension in your feet. Recall the tennis ball massage from page 39 in chapter 2 that demonstrated the fascial continuity between the sole of your foot and crown of your head. You can use those same instructions to gently stretch the fascia along your sole. The practice that follows will yield more specific results.

If you are one of the many people who have been told that you have flat feet, don't buy it. What you probably have are imbalanced and underactive feet. You can definitely improve this situation with the practices you're about to learn, with changes to your shoes, or both. Whether you have flat feet, high and rigid arches, or underactive toes, the following practices will help normalize your feet and balance your body above them.

Practice: Relaxing Your Arches

Stand so your tarsal sinuses are neither deeply indented nor flattened out. Place a tennis ball under the sole of your right foot, just beneath your tarsal sinus at the intersection of heel and arch. Distribute your weight on the ball so that you feel pressure through the tarsal sinus, not through your inner arch. Bend your right knee enough so that your hips can be level. Then steadily bend both knees farther, applying the weight of your body onto the ball. You may feel some discomfort as the tight fascia on the sole of your foot stretches. Hold the stretch for two slow breaths and then come up. Repeat the stretch four or five times.

When you remove the ball and stand flat on the floor, you'll likely have a distinct sensation that your heel is bigger on the foot that you worked. You may even feel that it extends farther behind you. These sensations contribute a feeling of support to your whole body. Repeat the exercise for the other foot.

Resist the temptation to save time by stretching both feet at once. Your feet and legs have individualize patterns. Correcting them requires giving them individual attention. After you've worked both feet with the ball, observe your stance again. The heightened sensations in your heels should allow your body to feel comfortable standing farther forward.

Where you find your balance on your feet has tremendous influence on your posture. Many people habitually stand with their weight centered over their heels. Having such a small base of support makes muscles on the front of the body tighten to prevent the body from falling backward. When you habitually stand on such a narrow base, you also shorten the postural muscles of your spine. This makes the back half of your body feel denser than the front. The added tension in the postural muscles acts like reins that hold your body back and increase the effort you must make to take a step forward.

With your balance over the whole of each foot, your body automatically moves into better orientation around its central axis. The foundation in your feet supports a more equal distribution of weight between the front and back portions of your body. It takes less muscular work to stay standing, and because your body is poised more forward over your feet, it takes less energy to get yourself going.

Your positioning over your feet even affects your breathing. When you habitually balance over your heels, the movement of breathing occurs primarily in the

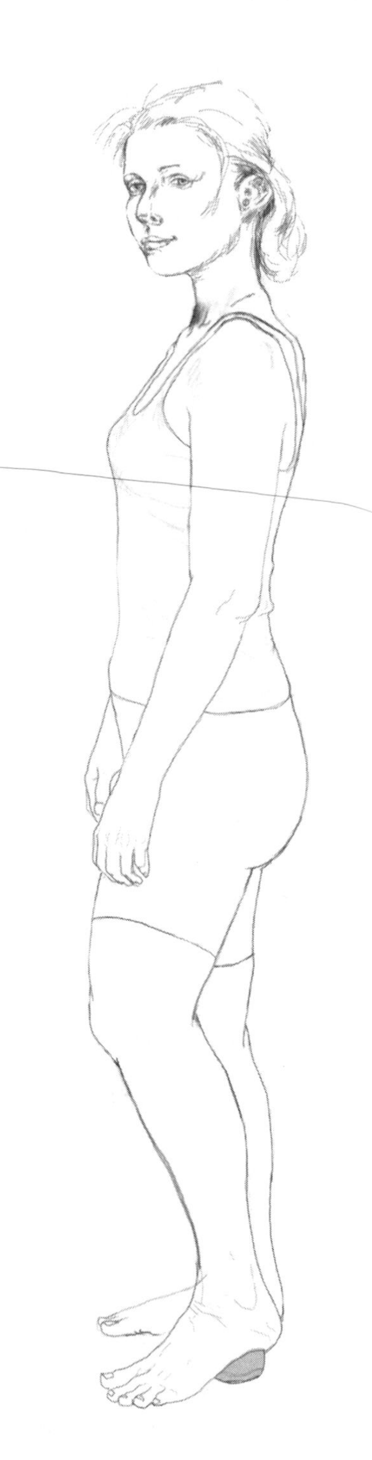

Fig. 7.2. To open and release the sole of your foot, place the ball just in front of your heel.

front of your rib cage. The excess tension of your back muscles blocks the rotation of your ribs where they meet the spine. With a better foundation in your feet, your breath can fill both the front and rear portions of your lungs.

Practice: Footprints on the Wall

This practice will help you open the joints of your feet so that the heels, arches, and toes can coordinate as they should in walking. It's a long exercise, with parts that should be practiced individually until you feel ready to combine them. Once you understand the exercise, you can practice the whole thing while you soak in the bathtub.

Lie on your floor or exercise mat and rest your feet on a wall. Have your thighs perpendicular to your torso and parallel to each other. Place your heels against the wall just above the level of your knees. (Glance down at your feet without lifting your head; you should be able to see your toes.) Place a folded towel beneath your neck and head for support if needed. Extend your arms out to the sides. Adjust your body until you can be comfortable. It should feel as though your soles are hanging on the wall; your thigh muscles should be relaxed. Breathe steadily and moderately. Relax your jaw and eyes.

Spread your toes and gently press the pad at the end of each toe into the wall. Try to press all ten toes equally, as if making toe prints on the wall. As your toes meld into the wall, stretch them out through the tips, lengthening the skin on the undersides of your toes. Try to give attention to each one of your toes. This will take time and patience.

As you work, keep the rest of your body in your awareness. Don't let the attention on your feet cause you to close any of your posture zones. Keep your pelvic floor spacious, especially the back triangle, and breathe continuously. Relax your hands, fingers, calves, and thighs. Move only your toes.

Practice: Opening Your Feet

The work with your toes will have brought the balls of your feet into firm contact with the wall. Equalize the pressure through the horizontal arch of your foot—from the ball of your little toe across to the ball of your big toe.

While keeping your toe pads and your horizontal arch melded into the wall, slightly reduce the pressure of your right heel. Relax it just enough so that you can stretch your heel down toward the floor, away from the ball of your foot. This action gives your midfoot a gentle traction. Next, carefully lengthen the left foot. Then, while maintaining firm contact through both forefeet, press both heels into the wall again. This should put you in touch with the fullness of your footprints. You may even feel some relaxation in your upper body as your feet open up.

Practice: Alternating Pressure between Forefoot and Heel

First, press more deeply into the wall with your heels while sustaining full skin contact with the balls of your feet and all ten toes. Then reverse the process: lighten the heel pressure and press more firmly through the forefoot. Alternate the pressure for several minutes, balancing out any disparity in the sensations of skin contact and pressure between your two feet.

Keep your thighs relaxed throughout the practice. Only your feet should be working. As you press through your forefoot, you may notice a faint sensation travel up through the fascia along the front of your body. You may feel it all the way up through your throat and into your face. As you press through your heels, look for sensation traveling up the back of your body to your skull. Come to rest with equal pressure between heels and forefeet.

Practice: Rocking from Stance Foot to Walking Foot

This practice uses the pronation and supination movements of your midfoot in relation to your heel. The heel itself should not move. Do the exercise one foot at a time at first.

With your toes elongated and the balls of your feet in firm contact with the wall, adjust your right heel to refresh the traction of your foot. Maintaining central pressure through your heel, increase the pressure into the balls of the fourth and fifth toes. There will be a tendency for your big toe to lift and be ungrounded as you move your midfoot into supination. To avoid this, keep the pad at the end of the big toe in firm contact with the wall. Then, slowly roll your foot across the horizontal arch toward the ball of the big toe. As your foot pronates, maintain steady pressure through your heel.

Relax, readjust your foot, reopen your posture zones, and begin again. After several rounds, switch to your left foot. Avoid pressing so hard into the wall that your back flattens into the floor. Preserve your neutral lumbar curve by opening the back triangle of your pelvic floor or by letting your pubic bone rest down. Keep your thighs relaxed and do not move your knees. Only your arches should be working. Time the movement of your feet with your breathing. This keeps you from holding your breath in concentration and helps you maintain a meditative pace.

To complete this practice, stand and take in the feeling of the changed relationship of your feet with the ground. As with the Relaxing Your Arches practice (p. 140), your weight will now be distributed over the entire surface of your feet, not just on the heels. This brings your central axis slightly forward and releases some load from your spine.

Exploration: Stepping into Your Whole Heel

The foot practices that you've done so far should have given you a new experience of the size of your heel—one third of your foot. When you walk, experiment with meeting the floor with the full surface of your heel rather than only its back edge. This will bring your central axis a bit forward as you move. Your body will stay centered over your feet, in contrast with the habit of stepping out with your heels and drawing your body up to meet them. The new pattern will not be possible, though, if you've closed your pelvic floor, lost inner corset support, or let your chest collapse.

If this way of walking feels contrived, forget about it for now. It may be that your hips cannot yet adapt to such a different use of your feet. It can help to review the Sacroiliac Rocking practice (p. 45); see also the box Sitting on a Ball (p. 60).

Bunions

A bunion is a painful enlargement of the joint at the base of the big toe. Bunions form in response to foot misalignment in which the big toe migrates toward the second toe. Although bunions tend to run in families, it is not the bunion that is passed from generation to generation but the faulty foot use. Bunions result when too much pressure is applied to the ball of the big toe during the push-off phase of walking. This happens if your knees and feet turn out, a pattern that often coincides with overpronation. If alignment of the feet and legs is not corrected, the twisting of the big toe worsens. Continued pressure stretches ligaments and tendons beyond their capacity to support the joint. In such a case, surgery may be necessary. The tendon of the big toe muscle *(flexor hallucis longus)* runs through a cleft in the ball of the big toe. In a severe bunion, this tendon twists free of its mooring. Having good tone in your big toe muscle can prevent this from happening. To activate the muscle, pay extra attention to keeping the pad of your big toe secure against the wall when you practice the Footprints on the Wall exercise.

Although a bunionectomy can remove the tissue accumulation that causes walking to be painful, it does not restore the ball of the foot to a healthy status. Postsurgical stiffness in the toe can lead to compensating imbalances and pain in your knee, hip, or spine. To keep this from happening to you, do everything you can to preserve the health of your toes. Your first line of defense against bunions is a sensible approach to selecting shoes. Nine out of ten bunions develop in women. Surely women's habit of squeezing their feet into shoes with pointed toes has something to do with this statistic.

If your big toe has begun to migrate toward your second toe, you need to activate your *abductor hallucis* muscle. The action of this tiny muscle, which lies long your inner arch between your heel and the base of your big toe, moves your big toe away from the others. The following practice will help you awaken this muscle.

Practice: Help for Bunions

While sitting so that you can see your foot on the floor, place a pencil a quarter-inch away from the side of your big toe. Keep your big toe pad in firm contact with the floor and slide your big toe sideways toward the pencil without lifting the toe off the floor. At first the only movement you make may be in you mind. Make several attempts and then rest.

As you attempt to widen your big toe cleavage, don't cheat by letting the small toes go in the opposite direction. Move only the big toe. Lightly massage your inner arch to bring awareness to the underused muscle. If you have a bunion, this practice will be maddeningly difficult. It can also result in a cramp in your abductor hallucis muscle. This is a signal that this muscle needs your attention. Massage the cramp away and begin again.

Persist with this practice for several months. Activation of your big toe muscles will change the function and feel of your foot even if the appearance of the bunion does not change.

Shoes and Insoles

Statistics show that the only thing that consistently stimulates someone to buy shoes is their appearance. But fashion trends are hardly good criteria if what you have been learning about your feet is true. For your feet to serve you long and well, your criteria should be whether the shoes provide a good foundation for healthy posture.

Rehabilitating your feet can be challenging. If you know that your feet are a liability but disciplined practice is not your style, you need to pay special attention to your shoes. Slip-on shoes make you lean back and scuff your feet, and although you're not conscious of doing it, you also contract foot muscles to keep the shoes on. This prevents your muscles from fully articulating your feet. Thong sandals can cause your big toe and second toe to squeeze together—a bunion in the making. They're also an especially poor choice for a long day at Disney World. Shoes with high, wedged soles reduce your foot's capacity to interact directly with the ground and make you susceptible to ankle injury.

Choose shoes with firm but flexible soles, a foot bed that feels good under your arches, and straps or laces that bind the shoe securely around your foot. For those who prefer to slip shoes on and kick them off quickly, a supportive shoe with Velcro straps offers almost the convenience of a slip-on shoe. The shoe should have a toe box that is broad enough to allow the ball of your foot to function like a hinge. Your toes should have room to spread and lengthen during push-off. When the toes are crowded together, the foot, and whole body, loses power in walking. Spend your shoe dollars on support and comfort rather than on style. If you must have your Manolo Blahnik spikes, save them for times when you won't be on your feet.

Supportive insoles for your shoes are an intelligent choice for those who overpronate. Sometimes generic inserts serve as well as expensive custom-made orthotics. Be sure that any insole you select is flexible enough to accommodate the motions of your feet in walking. The shoes or insoles should make your knees, back, and shoulders feel more relaxed. Research suggests that rigid orthotics actually weaken foot muscles, potentially making posture worse.*

Aligning Legs and Feet

Our knee joints are relatively straightforward hinges. Other than knee trauma, most imbalances in knees are due to poorly supportive feet or restricted motion in the hips. The orientation of the knees is usually determined by the rotation of the thighs, which, in turn, is influenced by the pelvis. If the pelvis is tilted back, the thighs, knees, and feet tend to turn outward when we are standing and walking. If the pelvis is tilted extremely forward, with an exaggerated lumbar curve, the thighs, knees, and feet tend to turn in. Although this is not true of everyone, these patterns are evident more often than not.

Imagine small light sources affixed to each of your kneecaps. Notice the direction of your "knee lights" as you walk. The beams can make parallel, inward- or outward-pointing paths. Ida Rolf, creator of Structural Integration, proposed that hips, knees, ankles, and "toe hinge" across the balls of the feet should function in perpendicular relationships to the body's central axis. Although Rolf's idea oversimplified the way the hip joint is used in walking, the exercises she prescribed work well for aligning your knees and ankles. One of these exercises follows.†

Practice: Aligning Your Legs

Aligning your legs is not as simple a process as having your car's wheels aligned, but it is every bit as necessary. This practice will put your legs in good order. To do it effectively requires attention to detail, but once it is mastered, you can do it while waiting for the toast to pop or standing in a checkout line.

Stand so that your feet are slightly farther apart than your sit bones. If you're used to a wider stance, this may feel confining. If so, relax your stance a bit, but have your feet no wider than your shoulders. Have your kneecaps facing forward, but don't force your feet into parallel alignment. (In time, the practice will bring your feet into a better relationship with your knees.) Release your pelvic floor, especially the back triangle. Stand so your weight feels evenly distributed over

*Several companies have developed shoes or shoe inserts intended to help the feet realign through tactile feedback. You'll find references in the appendix.

†Other Rolf Movement exercises for leg alignment are included in my book, *Balancing Your Body: A Self-help Approach to Rolfing Movement.*

your feet. Be aware of the fullness of your heels and the grounding through your toes, especially the pads of your big toes.

If you tend to overpronate, bring your awareness to your foot's outside arch. Find a stance that produces a medium-sized indentation in your tarsal sinus—not too deep, not too flat, but just right. If your arches are high and rigid, imagine your tarsal sinus becoming soft and open. Spread the skin on the soles of your feet as you did in the Footprints on the Wall exercise. Refresh the lift in your torso with healthy breathing and core support. Let your eyes gaze toward the horizon, and let the crown of your head ascend as if it were magnetized to the sky.

While sustaining the lift of your head, gradually and steadily move your shins forward. This will bend your hips, knees, and ankles. Lower your body only an inch or two. As you move, aim your "knee lights" over your second toes. Spend two breathing cycles making your descent. Then, slowly ascend by moving the crown of your head upward while pressing down through the soles of your feet. This action straightens your knees without overuse of your leg muscles.

Bend and straighten your knees several times, while patiently attending to the way your ankles, knees, and hips line up. As you move, let your awareness circulate between your upper body, legs, and pelvis. If you simply bend and straighten without remembering your whole body's alignment, the movement will not be therapeutic. By sustaining the lift of your head as you descend, you keep your joints spacious enough to allow a new coordination of your legs. (To facilitate leg alignment, review Wall Traction [p. 126]. In addition to stretching your shoulders, Wall Traction helps raise the weight of your torso off your legs and makes room for your hips, knees, and ankles to track with better alignment.)

If you're aware that your pelvis tilts backward, with your tail tucking under, you need to pay special attention to opening your anal triangle during this practice. To insure against tucking, place your fingertips under your two sit bones. As you move your knees forward, draw your sit bones slightly back and up with your fingers. Feel how this releases your thighs from your hip joints.

Notice the allocation of weight between your two feet. If you have more weight on one leg than the other, try to balance it out as you bend and straighten. You may experience a surprising shakiness in your legs as previously underused muscles are called into play. Relax between each attempt, allowing each time to be a fresh exploration of your legs. Hold the movements in your attention in a meditative way. Repatterning the deeply ingrained habits of grounding and balance cannot occur through a calisthenic mentality.

It can help to watch yourself in a mirror while you do this, but use the mirror only as a temporary guide. Sensing the new coordination of your legs is more important than seeing it.

Theresa's New Shoes

For Mother's Day, Carmen bought Theresa some expensive walking shoes, shoes her mother would never consider buying for herself. Theresa had protested for weeks before letting Carmen take her to the orthopedist. "There's nothing wrong with my knees," she said, "they're just old knees." The doctor agreed. "All the tests are negative," he told her. Take some aspirin; your knees are fine. But Carmen figured better support couldn't do Theresa's knees any harm, so she took a chance on the shoes.

Theresa's thriftiness made it hard to admit how good the shoes made her feel, and not just in her feet. "Taller" was the word that came to mind. Not only that, but in a few weeks she also forgot all about having elderly knees. She and little Rico could take much longer excursions. It was lovely to be able to keep up with her grandson.

SENTIENT FEET

In addition to being your physical foundation, your feet are perceptual organs. By orienting your body to the earth, your feet let you know where down is. Although obvious, this is something we do not always fully sense. The sole of each foot has more than seven thousand nerve endings that work together with countless sensors in the ankle joint for precise negotiation of your balance. Your feet, like your hands, are skintelligent. In a way that is similar to how sensation in your hands activates your serratus muscle, sensation in your feet stimulates the muscles of your inner corset. The following exploration will amplify the sensations in your feet.

EXPLORATION: SHIFTING SANDS

This exploration is a workout for the pressure and balance receptors in your soles and ankles. It will remind you of the Postural Sway exploration that you did in chapter 2. You're going to stand on a firm couch cushion or yoga bolster with your eyes closed. For security, place the bolster within arm's distance of a wall.*

Simply stand on the bolster, allowing your body to adjust to the subtle shifts in your balance. Rather than trying to control your balance, let your feet receive impressions from the mobile surface. Allow your body to move in response to those impressions. Feel your feet negotiating your relationship with gravity. Feel the shifting and reorienting of your vertical axis.

Keep relaxing any tensions that creep into your shins, calves, and thighs. Release any closure of your core, hands, or breath. Relax your eyes—they can be tense even when they're closed. Stand on the bolster for three minutes before reading on.

When you step down from the bolster, notice any change in your perception of the ground. For many of you, the ground will feel more "there"—more substantial or trustworthy. Your body, too, may feel more substantial, more present. These perceptions have enormous influence on your posture. Savor and memorize them.

If you feel that you lack grounding, practice this exploration daily to restore your connection to the earth. Some of you may find that the practice has a surprisingly emotional effect. How we connect to the earth—how we ground, support, and balance ourselves—affects our hearts and minds as well as our bodies.

---

*Many fitness and physical therapy programs use wobble boards to challenge balance. Such surfaces are too unstable for the kind of perceptual repatterning being undertaken in this exploration.

Pushing and Reaching

In chapter 6, we saw that gestures of reaching out correlate with our orientation to our surroundings. We can reach out with hands, heart, mouth, eyes, or even feet. In a similar way, the action of pushing helps us orient ourselves to the material world. Pushing is one of our first actions as human beings. We push our way through the birth canal with our feet. It could even be said that being able to push effectively empowers us to reach out.

To push effectively, we need to sense the thing we're pushing against. As you experienced in chapter 6, we do not always feel what we are touching. By the same token, we often push without feeling. Yet, as Alison experienced in Home Depot with her shopping cart, pushing something is easier when we engage our skintelligence.

To experience how this affects your feet, review Aligning Your Legs (p. 147), in the following way: While bending your knees, let the skin of your soles be as open to the ground as they were when you stood on an unstable surface. Imagine that your feet are in contact with something that has life. To rise, press your feet more deeply into that living floor. Let the pressure drive your body upward, thrusting the crown of your head closer to the sky.

When you push with feeling, straightening your knees results from the push of your feet, not from effort in your knees. This is an efficient way to use your legs because it reduces the work of your thigh muscles. From now on, incorporate the downward push into your leg alignment practice.

Exploration: Sitting to Standing

The action of moving from sitting to standing offers you many opportunities to practice your new awareness of pushing the ground with your feet. Start from healthy sitting. Feel your feet, including all ten toes, in contact with the floor. Open your soles to the earth.

Lean forward from your hips as if reaching forward for something. At the instant when your heart is directly over your feet, push them down into the floor. Imagine your feet are coated in ink so that as you push down, you make an indelible impression. You can also imagine the floor is made of soft wet sand so that as you push, you leave an indentation. The pushing action also thrusts your head skyward. Play this out several times. Your feet push down to let your head and heart ascend. The action is a duality of downward and upward movements, of simultaneous grounding and motion into space.

Exploration: Pushing the Floor

Remind yourself of Two-way Touching (p. 132), in which you did a household task with skintelligence. Vacuuming was suggested, but sweeping, washing windows, or polishing the car work just as well. Try it again. Open your soles to perceive the ground in the same way that you open your hands to sense the tool you are using. Instead of just standing still and pushing your hand into the task, let the action begin from your feet. You can push your feet down to propel the broom handle or polishing cloth in the same way that you pushed down to propel your body from sitting to standing. Your work becomes a marriage of pushing and reaching.

Grounding

Your feet can't support your posture if they don't sense the ground. When feet and legs are tense, perception of the ground fades along with accompanying feelings of support, security, and balance. If you don't fully feel the ground, you will seek support elsewhere—in your pelvic floor, gut, breath, shoulders, or jaw. Closure in any posture zone restricts movement throughout your body. Your posture can't be adaptable, or your movement graceful, without sentient feet.

Early in this chapter, you noticed your body's response when you imagined walking on an ice-cold floor. Similar tensions result when we hurry or try to walk without making any noise. Firm footing also diminishes when we fantasize about the future or are distracted by the past. Sensitive feet help anchor us in the here and now. The following practice will invite you to attune your feet to the earth.

Practice: Sacred Ground

As you walk, shift your attention so that you become aware of your feet being touched by the ground as well as touching it. Imagine the floor coming up to meet your feet and welcoming them. Let your soles, ankles, and shins relax and become open to impressions from the ground. Feel the floor in your ankles as you walk. Sense your impact with the floor in your shins. Feel it in your knees and hip joints.

Alison's Success

Alison was amazed at how little effort she needed for vacuuming as long as she paid attention to her hands and feet. It actually felt energizing to let her legs do the work.

"That skin trick," she thought, "it's magic." She had the feeling that her legs were driving her spine and that her spine gave power to her shoulders and elbows. That left her hands free to steer the vacuum around the furni-

ture. Her chest stayed expansive. You'd almost have thought vacuuming was her favorite sport.

Walking felt different, too, as if the ground itself were softer. It helped to remember that her feet were springs instead of bricks. Alison felt so good that she decided to attempt cleaning the chandelier again. She had her "aha" the moment she climbed onto the stool. It was wobbly. She could only manage the instability by trusting her feet. Before, she'd been trying so hard to center herself that she'd lost her foundation. Now she could reach up and scrub to her heart's content. When the stool wobbled, she opened her feet instead of closing her pelvic floor. As if rewarding her for her patience, the antique chandelier reluctantly revealed a design of enameled roses.

Healing posture is a process of accumulating a new repertoire of sensations. By patiently cultivating healthy sensations in your posture zones, you feed your reptilian brain the information it needs to construct healthy new habits. If you use your analytical brain to "have good posture" or "walk right," you will only block the smooth coordination that your brain stem can provide. The result will feel awkward and inauthentic. So take your time with this book. Backtracking to practices in earlier chapters can deepen your experience of healthy posture.

The next chapter concludes your tour of the healthy posture zones. Exploration of the head will complete your list of resources for relating your grasp of things, ideas, and people to an open yet contained and supported stance.

8 FACING THE WORLD

Appearance is temporary. It's nothing you can rely on. In the end, gravity always wins.

JOHNNY DEPP

Mika streamlines her way across the parking lot, feet grazing the asphalt, arms hugging her sides. Her gaze is fixed in midair about eight feet ahead. She notices nothing to her right or left—not the sun glinting off cars or the pastel wash of the morning sky. She ignores the fragile breeze that brushes against her skin. What she sees is the day ahead, the quarterly reports, the lunchtime conference, the . . .

She stops, aware that she's holding her breath. Again! She fights the urge to gulp air through her mouth. "Low, slow, moderate," she mutters to herself. It's so much easier to breathe right when she's at home practicing. She loves how her tummy disappears when her inner corset turns on. She's walking again, more upright for the moment.

Her doctor says there's nothing wrong—her headaches, her trouble sleeping. She just needs to relax more. So it's all in her head? Stepping up her pace, she enters the building. There's Roger. What about that report he promised? "Hey, Roger . . ."

Mika is not alone in getting ahead of herself. Like many people, she harbors tensions within her face and skull that rebound throughout her body and manifest as habits she can't seem to change. Her problem is twofold. She not only loses her orientation in space but she also tries to stabilize herself with the part of her body intended for perception.

A Natural Phenomenon

In the introduction to this book, you read: "The essence of posture, then, is the unique way in which each of us negotiates between moving and holding still in relationship to gravity." As we approach our last healthy posture zone, let's review how the previous chapters have fleshed out that statement.

Conventional rules for improving posture position the flesh around a static plumb line and train the body to move from that imposed center. If, instead, we follow the new rules of posture, we will regard the body's central axis as a dynamic manifestation of the process of orienting to gravity and the world outside our bodies. By the new rules, the gravitational plumb line is a dynamic perceptual activity, not just a position in space. Orientation is ongoing. It proceeds from moment to moment as long as we are awake. The gravity line is dynamically expressed within our selves. It is symbolic of our stance between the earth and the heavens.

The central axis is the reference point for the stabilizing actions that let us move our limbs to interact with the world. The posture zones are places where habitual stabilization can either restrain or emancipate that axis. The zones act like valves that open or close the central line. Our bodies should be free to sink and rise through each zone as we make our way from moment to moment. Through the activities in the preceding chapters, you have felt how the sensitive interaction of your feet with the ground improves your posture. You've noticed how your stance and walking benefit from an open pelvis and how the steady, mild closure in the lower abdomen secures the lower spine. You've understood that breathing creates both ascent and surrender and that gestures of work and love should grant the spine a skyward thrust.

How adaptably we express our postural orientations to earth and sky is a reflection of our histories—our responses to the traumas, however slight or great, that have made us wince, collapse, or stiffen. When sedentary lifestyles collude with hurt to curl us inward, we invert our natural polarity and lose our relationship with both ground and surroundings. With the central line imploded, our bodies can neither fully expand with joy and power, nor yield with ease or grace.

Now, we arrive at our uppermost posture zone. As the platform for the senses that negotiate balance, the head can complete our ascent or block it. The orienting senses help us relate to our surroundings and complement our relationship with the earth. This chapter explores what happens to posture and movement when we attempt to stabilize ourselves through the zone designed for knowing where we are.

Balance

Our bodies have three interacting neurological mechanisms that keep us balanced around our plumb lines: our eyes relate us to our surroundings, the inner ear rights our heads relative to gravity's pull, and pressure and balance receptors in our feet connect us to the ground.

Recall the Shifting Sands exploration (p. 149), in which you stood on a bolster to activate the receptors in your soles and ankles. When you closed your eyes to increase the stimulation of your feet, you also were activating the balance mechanism of your inner ear. Information from the feet is combined in the brain with information from the inner ear. Nerves to the inner ear are fully developed before birth—an indication of the primary importance of the sense of balance. We are equipped to deal with gravity even before we are born.

For most people, vision is the primary orienting sense. When our eyes dominate the other senses, the sensory acuity of our feet fades. This erodes our foundations and makes us overstabilize in other zones. The work of this chapter is to release tensions in the head and neck that undermine the natural cooperation of your eyes, feet, and inner ears. Such tensions are usually misplaced attempts to stabilize your body.

Anatomy: Temporal Bone, Mandible, and Suboccipital Muscles

If you cover your ears with your palms, your thumbs will be on the base of your skull, your *occiput.* Your palms and fingers will lie across your *temporal bones,* and the heels of each hand will rest on the angle of your jaw, your *mandible.*

Your temporal bone is the skeletal portal of your inner ear. The temporal bone and mandible interact at the *temporal mandibular joint—TMJ* for short. To locate this joint, lightly place two fingers directly in front of your ears and open and close your mouth.

The muscles that open and close your jaw pull on the skull and the neck vertebrae. Strain in the jaw muscles is transferred to your neck and relays down your throat into your shoulders, diaphragm, and pelvic floor. Jaw tension can also transmit strain to the temporal bone and inner ear, interfering with balance.

The joint between the base of your skull and first cervical vertebra (the *atlanto-occipital joint*) is shaped to allow the front-to-back nodding that Western culture interprets as "yes." It also allows a side-to-side wobble that we understand as "maybe," but other cultures use to communicate affirmation, pleasure, or defiance. The first neck vertebra pivots around the second to allow the rotation that almost universally expresses the concept of "no."

Your expressive head motions are made by tiny muscles known as the *suboccipitals,* which connect the base of your skull to your upper two neck vertebrae. These muscles lie underneath your trapezius and other larger neck muscles. The suboccipitals have more motion sensors than any other part of the body, which gives them an important role to play. When you stood on the bolster earlier, the balance sensors of your inner ears received information about the changing pressures under your feet. While your inner ear helped keep your head upright, the suboccipitals kept your head aligned with your body.

Because of fascial links between your face and neck, any tension in your jaw, nose, or eyes can harden and immobilize the suboccipital muscles, undermining your balance and preventing healthy posture.

To sense your suboccipital muscles, lightly place your finger pads just below the base of your skull at the back of your neck. Rest your fingers as lightly as a butterfly. Then, imagine that you are watching a fly buzzing

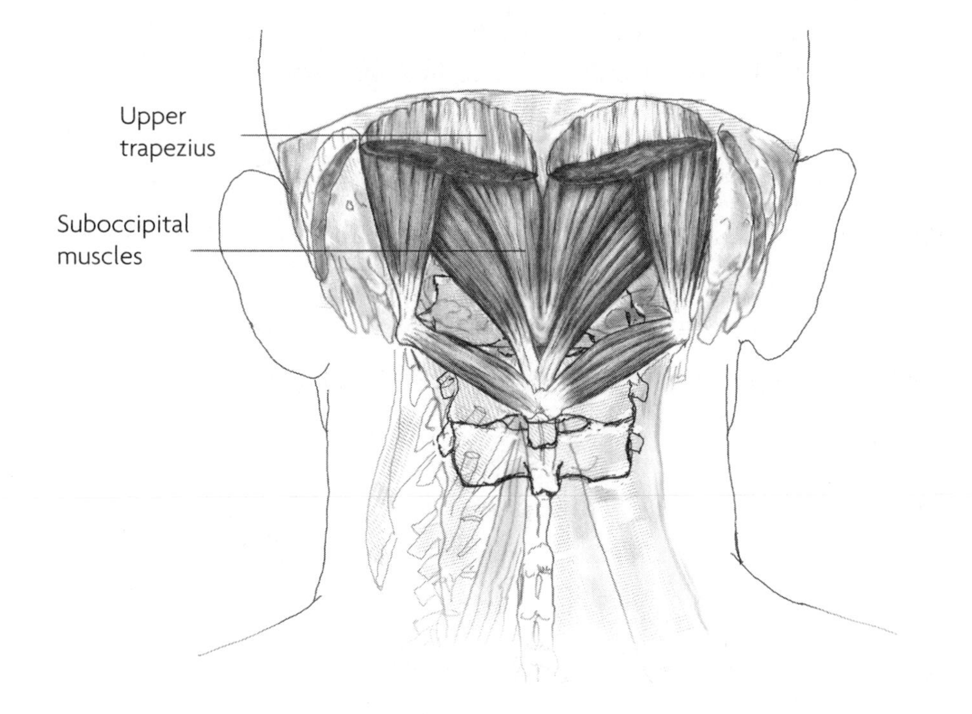

Fig. 8.1. The tiny suboccipital muscles keep your head aligned with your body as you move about.

around in front of you. Move only your eyes, not your head. As your eyes track the insect—up, down, around in circles—you can feel your suboccipitals at work.

For contrast, narrow your focus as if staring hard at a computer screen. Furrow your brow and purse your lips as if struggling to understand something. You'll feel the suboccipitals harden. Notice what this does to your breathing, shoulders, and core.

The anatomy of the region between your jaw and skull, or *cranium,* is complex. The fascial connections between the floor of your mouth and the base of your cranium form a horizontally oriented valve-like structure that can impinge on the central gravity line. When tension in your face locks up the suboccipitals, the strain travels down your spine all the way to your sacrum. You felt this in chapter 2, when you tensed your jaw and were unable to smoothly rock your sacrum (Holistic Impact, p. 48). Tension around your sacrum prevents your feet from meeting the ground securely. So, healthy functioning of the three balancing systems—eyes, ears, and feet—depends on the responsiveness of your suboccipital muscles.

Facial Tensions

The following explorations will help you become acquainted with tensions that you might be harboring in your face. When you meet a tension that seems familiar, adopt that exploration as a healthy posture practice.

Exploration: Jaw and Tongue Tensions

While sitting comfortably, trace your mandible with your fingertips, starting just in front of your ears and following around the angle of your jaw to your chin. Get a sense of what a substantial bone it is. Open your mouth slightly and let your mandible hang slack for a few moments. Appreciate its distinct presence, separate from the rest of your head. Feel its weight.

Then close your lips gently, leaving space between your upper and lower back molar teeth and retaining your sense of the mandible's weight. Touch your lips together so lightly that you can't be sure whether they are touching. Soften the floor of your mouth. Appreciate how large the inside of your closed mouth can be when you relax your jaw.

The suggestions in the previous paragraphs will help you relax your temporal mandibular joint. Typically, this makes the cheeks feel longer or fuller than usual. Compare this sensation with the way your jaw usually feels. Notice whether it affects your throat or chest.

Now, become aware of your tongue. Allow it to be flat and broad at the root. Let it rest like a puddle along the floor of your mouth. Notice how relaxing your tongue affects your throat and your breathing. Because the mouth opens into your lungs and digestive tract, tension in your jaw or tongue can relay down through your respiratory and digestive core. Feel what occurs internally when your tongue assumes a different shape or presses against the roof of your mouth.

Exploration: Nose and Palate Tension

The roof of your mouth—your *hard palate*—is located just in front of the place where your skull meets your neck. Easing tension in this region is beneficial for your neck and whole spine.

Lie on a carpeted floor or exercise mat and support your head and neck with a folded towel. Allow your throat to be soft and open, the way it feels just after you've swallowed. Remind yourself of the healthy breathing practices. When you breathe, your palate naturally changes shape. It widens with inhalation and narrows with exhalation as the bones and fascia of your skull accommodate to changing pressures. Focusing on this motion helps you relax your head.

As you inhale, imagine that your upper back molars are moving ever so slightly outward toward your cheekbones. As you exhale, let your palate relax. These suggestions soften and widen the area deep behind your nostrils and let you receive your inhalation into the root of your nose. This, in turn, helps relax your suboccipital muscles. Releasing the palate relaxes the eyes by giving them a broader platform on which to rest. It can also transmit a sense of ease down through your jaw, throat, shoulders, and even your belly.

For contrasting sensations, sniff your breath in through the front of your nostrils. Notice how doing this narrows the roof of your mouth and tightens the muscles at the base of your skull. You'll also feel a different response in your rib cage.

Once you have experienced the broad feeling across your palate and the open feeling at the root of your nose, practice sustaining these sensations while

Mouth Breathing Revisited

Too little tone in your jaw muscles can be as problematic as too much. When watching TV, listening to a lecture, or concentrating on computer work, notice whether your mouth is ajar and whether you are breathing through it. Be aware of sensation in your inner corset when you are mouth breathing.

In clinical practice, it has been observed that laxity of the jaw and inner corset often coincide, contributing to a vicious circle of inadequate core support and anxiety-producing breathing patterns. In such cases, the crura of the diaphragm may be recruited to stabilize the core, making matters worse. To heal the relationship between your jaw and core, combine the awareness gained in this chapter with the practices in chapters 4 and 5.

you're upright. The relaxation produced by this simple awareness can do wonders for your posture, and for your state of mind.

EXPLORATION: JAW AND INNER EAR

Lie on your back with your neck supported. You can have your legs extended or your knees bent. Roll your head very slowly to the right while letting your tongue and lower jaw follow the movement of your head. As your face turns to the right, feel your mandible settling to that side. Feel your tongue and the flesh of your cheek melting toward the floor.

Take one full breathing cycle to make the turn and a second cycle to roll your head, jaw, and tongue back to center, Your tongue and jaw may try to lead the motion of your head. Teach yourself to let them follow.

To deepen the relaxation of your jaw, imagine softening your inner ear on the side to which you are turning. Alternate rolling your head to each side several times. The tenser your jaw is, the more time and patience will be required to release it. When your jaw is relaxed, your whole body will likely feel more grounded and open. Breathing may seem to flow deeper into the chest and your shoulders and arms will relax their grip.

Ty's Miracle

Remember Ty—the boy with his hands soldered to the Xbox and his eyes glued to the TV screen? He now seems to have traded in his obsession with computer games for an obsession with basketball. What a change! His mom just can't figure it out. All of a sudden, her son is polite! He's nice to his little brother. And all that weight he'd gained drinking sodas on the couch? Well, the pounds just melted right off. It had to be a miracle!

Ty, if he thought about it, might say that his head doesn't feel pinched any more. Every time the orthodontist tightened his braces, it felt like his skull was in a vise. The only way he could drown out the pain was with video games. With the braces off now, his teeth feel light. His whole body feels light. He doesn't even remember the chest pain that kept him off the basketball court.

Your Mobile Skull

Until the twentieth century, Western science assumed that the joints between the twenty-one bones of the cranium were immobile. In the 1920s, an osteopathic physician discovered a faint, rhythmic motion in the skull. The motion reflects the flow of the cerebrospinal fluid that bathes the brain and spinal cord. It can be felt because of the elasticity of the sutures between the cranial bones.

A therapy method based in osteopathic techniques rebalances the hydraulic pressures within the skull and spinal cord. By restoring harmony to the nervous system in this way, CranioSacral Therapy can relieve problems such as headaches, ringing in the ears, TMJ pain, emotional issues, and learning problems.*

In Ty's case, tension created by the braces inhibited the inherent motion of his cranial bones. This, in turn, upset his personality.† His mouth breathing was an attempt to accommodate the dental appliances and relieve the strain they created in his jaw.

Many of us harbor stabilizing tensions in our jaws, eyes, and suboccipital muscles. Tension in the head tightens muscles and fascia that lie over the skull and makes the scalp feel like a bathing cap that's way too tight. Such tension blocks normal cranial motion.

Exploration: Distinguishing Cranium and Face

Apart from our hairstyles, most of us have little awareness of the back of our heads. We rely on our faces to orient ourselves. To experience a different use of your head and neck, mentally divide your head into front and back halves. Call everything in front of your ears "face" and everything behind "head." Sitting with healthy posture, experiment with turning your head from the back of your skull. Look right by moving the back of your head left. Look up by moving the back of your head down. Look down by letting the back of your cranium ascend. Spend several minutes looking around in this manner.

For a contrasting sensation, turn your head by moving your face. You'll notice that your neck and head jut slightly forward when you do it this way. You may also feel that the movements are less smooth. Your head weighs ten to twelve pounds. Displacing your head in front of your chest adds significantly to the weight your neck and shoulders must carry. Neck and shoulder tension are the inevitable result.

*Refer to the appendix for more information about CranioSacral Therapy.

†Some orthodontists and dentists have become aware of the holistic impact of dental work. Consult the appendix for references.

Tension in your neck, especially in the suboccipitals, increases tension throughout your body.

When you give attention to the back of your head, you bring the muscles in the front and back of your neck into better balance. The suboccipitals can relax a bit. The resulting lift of your head decompresses your neck vertebrae, improving their mobility. It also improves your posture and breathing.

To complete this exploration, try to feel the play of motion down through your spine to your sacrum as you look around from the back of your cranium. Be sure that you're sitting well when you do this. If you slouch, you won't be able to sense the connection between your head and lower body.

The Eyes and Vision

For many of you, moving from the face probably felt familiar and was accompanied by a sense of reaching out with the eyes. Regardless of how well you see, you can use your eyes in various ways. Your focus can be tight or diffuse. Your vision can be strained or receptive. None of these necessarily affect your visual acuity, but they all affect your posture. The following explorations will help you experience how your visual sense affects your body.

Exploration: Narrow Focus and Open Focus

Stand with healthy posture and a good foundation in your feet. As you breathe moderately and steadily through your lower ribs, seek balance between the front and back of your body.

Observe some detail in the room, such as a doorknob or a light switch. Train your eyes on the object with the intent of finding out as much about it as you can. Study it. Analyze it. Notice what happens in the rest of your body as you do this. Especially notice your suboccipitals and your breathing. As your eyes reach out to grasp the object, you might even feel tension in your hands, as if they are very subtly grasping, too.

Now, deliberately soften your focus so that you see nothing in particular but instead notice all the colors and shapes surrounding you. Feel your body's response as you do this—how it seems to make you lose your relationship to the ground. It may even blur your sense of your body's boundaries.

Renew your stance and restore your breathing. This time find a partnership between these two types of vision. Look again at the same object but sustain your peripheral vision at the same time. Notice that your breathing becomes more relaxed and that your posture can remain open.

Appreciate any differences in your perception of the object. Chances are that you see it as clearly as before but you now see it in relation to its surroundings. Perhaps a play of light across the doorknob makes you aware of wind rustling the trees outside the open door.

How we use our eyes reflects our culture and lifestyles. Studies show that people from holistically oriented Asian cultures move their eyes between the foreground and background of a scene. Their eyes naturally seek a relationship between a subject and its context. In contrast, goal-oriented Westerners tend to focus on the most colorful or most rapidly moving object in a scene.

Reptile Vision and Balance

Peripheral vision is linked to your subcortical brain, which is also the part of your brain that automatically organizes your movements. However, when your eyes focus tightly, you are using the cortical brain and this interferes with your coordination. An experiment will make this clear. Narrow your focus to stare at an object while you stand on one leg. Try to maintain your balance by using your eyes to grasp the object in front of you. Do your best to control your balance. Notice the efforts of your legs and feet as you do this.

Now, relax your eyes and legs for a moment. Remind the soles of your feet to sense the temperature and texture of the floor. Then, using your eyes to see peripherally as well as what's in front of you, stand again on the same leg. Forget about trying to balance. Focus instead on the skin on the sole of your foot. Feel that foot in full contact with the floor as you extend your visual awareness to your sides and back as well as forward.

If you expand your vision before you assume the one-legged stance, you'll notice it is easier to find your balance and keep it. Because peripheral vision is tied to your subcortical brain, engaging it automatically controls your balance. When you tightly focus your vision, your analytical brain assumes control of your body, but it can't compute sensations and direct movements fast enough to keep you balanced. Without reflexive intelligence from your subcortical brain centers, your body seeks stability by engaging muscles that harden and close your posture. Thus, when you diminish the spatial dimension of your vision, you also compress the space within your joints.

The following explorations help you release eye tension caused by habitually narrowed focus.

Exploration: Releasing Eye Tension

Lie on a carpeted floor or exercise mat and support your head and neck with a folded towel. You'll be working with your eyes closed, so read through the instructions before you begin.

Imagine your eye sockets deepening to let your eyes rest into the back of your head. Soften the inner and outer corners of your eyes. Soften your eyelids and eyelashes. Sense the weight of your eyes as they rest back into their sockets.

Roll your head slowly to the right by moving the back of your head to the left, taking one full breathing cycle to make the turn. As your head turns, let your closed eyes roll within their sockets, following the movement of your face. Soften the outer corner of your right eye and the inner corner of your left eye so that both eyes can rest more deeply to the right. Take another breathing cycle to return your head and eyes to center. Feel the weight of the back of your head drawing your eyes back home. Your eyes will try to anticipate the action, so you need to make sure that they follow the motion of your head.

Repeat your head roll to the other side. Take plenty of time with this exercise. When your eyes feel softer, open them and sit up. Let your eyes remain soft and deep in their sockets as you look around, moving from the back of your head. You'll notice that having relaxed eyes makes it easier to receive peripheral impressions. If you work at a computer, you will benefit from doing this at least once each day. You can do it while sitting at your desk.

Exploration: Receptive Eyes

Notice how the way you use your eyes affects your posture when you walk. Move toward a goal with tightly focused intent. For example, you might cross the room to pick up your car keys. Notice your overall sensations of tension or ease. Notice sensations of openness or closure in your posture zones.

Contrast those feelings with how you feel while walking toward the same object but allowing your eyes to take in your surroundings. Be aware of colors and shapes washing past you as you move through the space. Feel the caress of the air over your skin. Compare the ease and mobility of this walk to the previous one. When you walk with two-way vision, you can see where you're headed while also remaining aware of where you are.

When you engage your peripheral vision and focused vision simultaneously, your eyes become receptive. You can cultivate receptive vision while you're reading. Let yourself remain aware of your environment while your eyes scan the words. When you look at anything in this manner, your eyes remain soft, the way they felt after doing the Releasing Eye Tension exploration (p. 164).

If you have a habit of overfocusing with your eyes, you'll need to practice two-way vision on a consistent basis. Designate specific places or times in your daily routine as reminders to notice how you're using your eyes. As you do, you may experience some interesting shifts in your outlook.

Just as you can touch and be touched by the tools of daily living, you also can let your eyes simultaneously seek and receive what you see. Two-way use of your eyes contributes spatial dimension to your posture. In contrast, intense and narrow focus not only compresses your body but also diminishes your sense of personal presence.

Eye Level

Like many people, you might have a habit of gazing at the floor when walking, even though seeing where the feet are being put is rarely necessary. When you do this, your neck bends forward to follow your eyes. Then, to reduce strain on your neck, your chest drops, distorting your breathing. This is a prime example of how closure in one posture zone cascades into closure in another.

Looking down can be a way to achieve privacy or to disconnect from other people. Although privacy can be at a premium in a crowded world, it's better to find it without sacrificing your orientation. If the habit of looking down sounds familiar, two-way vision is an important practice for you. When you're walking, let your gaze be level with the horizon. When you need to glance down, as in navigating steps or a rocky trail, momentarily tip your head without rounding your shoulders and jutting your neck forward.

If you should find yourself feeling uncomfortable moving through a crowd, practice being aware of the spaces between things. Focus on what artists call negative space. By maintaining your spatial orientation in this way you can keep an open posture and still get where you're going.

Mika Loses Her Grip

Mika has been making progress in changing how she uses her body at work. She had been "white-knuckling" her computer's mouse. When she remembers to handle it with her skin instead of her muscles, her arm automatically relaxes. The breath of relief that follows reminds her to readjust her sitting. So far, so good.

But lately she's noticed that her eyes grip the monitor as tightly as her hand was gripping the mouse. She has an idea. What if she keeps just 5 percent of her attention on the fact that there's space between herself and the screen? There's the screen—the words and the numbers—and here she is, sitting two feet away. No need to "eye-grab" at the screen if she's that close, now is there?

She feels better. By not letting the computer imprison her eyes, she prevents it from invading her personal space. That makes her feel more open all over, as if she has more space between the bones in her arms, space between her ribs, space everywhere. People would think she was nuts if they could read her thoughts.

She tries her new trick in the parking lot after work. Letting her eyes softly receive her surroundings seems to make the ground feel firmer under her feet. Fascinated by this phenomenon, she takes a detour around the lot just to enjoy the unique sensations in her feet.

Ordinarily Mika would have mentally driven away before she even opened the car door. Today she feels calm, as if the universe has just offered her more time.

Exploration: Welcoming the World

In this exploration you will work with the relationship between a relaxed orientation of your head and neck and expressive use of your arms. Begin by establishing healthy standing posture—ground your feet, open and stabilize your core, and relax your hands. Soften your eyes, nostrils, lips, tongue, and jaw. Be aware of your surroundings. Then extend your arms and hands in front of you in a gesture of welcome.

Notice the difference when you make the same gesture while doing any of the following: narrowing your focus, pressing your tongue to your upper palate, pursing your lips, or breathing through the front of your nose. When you induce tension in your head in any of these ways, the gesture of your arms will feel less welcoming. Using your eyes, tongue, or jaw to stabilize your head diminishes your sense of personal space. In so doing, it also limits your capacity for expression.

A Sense of Space

Our ears and eyes inform us about our surroundings. When we learn to relax any unconscious tensions within the head, our orienting senses are better able to organize posture. Spatial orientation is the source of postural lift and the antidote to gravity's downward pull. Without a sense of space, we'd stay flattened to the ground, unaware of our potential to move. We stand and walk in response to "what's out there," which we can know about only through our senses.

When you grasp the world with your eyes or when tension in the jaw interferes with the delicate balancing of your head by your suboccipital muscles, you misuse your head to stabilize yourself. This diminishes your perception of space. Then, because you have an inadequate sense of support from your surroundings, you seek stability by closing down somewhere along your centerline.

Our perception of spatial dimensions affects our relationships as well as our bodies. This includes relationships with activities, ideas, and people. Most of us know how it feels to merge with an interesting or pressing task to the point of losing self-awareness. At such times we may overwork, making mistakes and harming our bodies in the process. When we concentrate too hard on solving mental problems, our worried thoughts leave no space for new ideas to arise.

Losing a sense of space between yourself and another person can make a relationship feel so intense that your awareness of personal ground and space may be lost. Merging with another is natural between mother and infant and during sexual intimacy between bonded partners, but it can be immobilizing in other contexts. Freedom to move within a relationship requires not only that we sustain our personal ground and sense of space but also that we acknowledge the space between ourselves and the other person.

Moving Ahead

Driving home in a sudden downpour, Mika feels her body hardening. The highway is slick and drivers are reckless. A vague pain at the base of her skull reminds her to stop peering so intently through the windshield. When she lets her peripheral vision kick in, her eyes relax and the headache evaporates. She stops craning her neck and even lightens her grip on the steering wheel. A big sigh reveals that she was holding her breath—again—and pressing her tongue hard against the back of her palate. She'd been trying to stabilize her eyes with her tongue.

Healthy posture keeps eluding Mika. The more she opens one posture zone, the more another one seems to close. Perhaps you've had similar experiences.

Mika now has good awareness of how she stabilizes herself with respect to her own center. She gradually understands more about how her orientation to the world around her affects her body. But there are so many old and new sensations to feel—it's a lot to take in.

Habits take a long time to develop, so it's unreasonable to expect them to change overnight. As Alfredo told her months ago, Mika needs to relax. She'll get nowhere trying to juggle every new awareness at once or beating herself up whenever an old habit recurs. Besides, since all six posture zones are linked through the fascial system, making a change in even one area improves her posture overall.

It will help Mika, and you, to more fully understand how stability and orientation affect walking, exercise, and other activities. The next part—"Motion"—will help you put it all together.

PART FOUR

MOTION

There is nothing you can do without moving.

TWYLA THARP

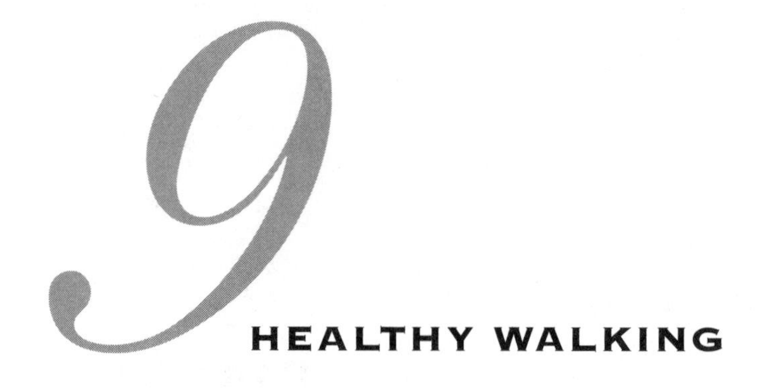

HEALTHY WALKING

I'm not a passenger,
I am the ride.

CHRIS SMITHER,
FOLKSINGER

Ever since she caught a demoralizing glimpse of herself in a plate glass window, Mika has been trying to figure out how to walk. She studies how people at work are walking and how movie stars walk in movies. Nobody looks graceful except dancers, and then only when they're dancing. But tonight she thinks she's found it—the perfect walk. She's so excited that she's invited her neighbor Alfredo over to see it.

"It's a documentary about women in Africa," she tells him. "Their lives seem unbearably difficult. But take a look at just this one part." She flicks on the DVD player.

A woman strides along a dirt road, her broad bare feet stirring puffs of dust. A corner of her colorful skirt flickers in the morning breeze and her bracelets tinkle and sparkle in the sun. She balances a bundle of sticks on her head.

"I read somewhere that an elephant's feet hear vibrations in the earth," says Mika. "It's how they communicate. See, Alfredo, her feet look like they can hear things too."

The woman's pelvis has a sensual sway and her hips softly cushion the impact of her steps. Her hips seem to blend the motions of her legs and spine into an undulating wave. Her chest and shoulders are open and generous, her breasts and belly borne with womanly pride. The woman's whole body seems to be in sentient communication with both land and heavens. Occasionally she laughs aloud as if with pleasure in her own sheer physicality.

"She's like living water," says Alfredo, "and the sticks are floating on her head."

"Can we ever learn to walk this way?"

Posture in Motion

Your walk is your posture in motion. Now that you've learned to minimize unnecessary tension in your body through the healthy use of your posture zones, you're ready to embrace a healthier way of moving. Changing your walk lets you sustain the improvements to your posture. On an average day, you take about ten thousand steps. If you spend a day at Disney World, you double that number. The more your steps embody healthy posture, the healthier your posture becomes.

We will begin our exploration of walking with a closer look at the way your perceptions color your relationship with gravity. You'll discover that you have a preferred way to orient your body before you take a step, and that this perceptual preference influences your habitual gait. By cultivating unfamiliar perceptions, you'll discover the grace that is hidden beneath your old habits. In the second part of the chapter, you'll discover the anatomical logic that underlies healthy walking. When your walking is in harmony with your structural design, it becomes both efficient and beautiful. Grace is built in. You need only to get out of the way and let it happen.

Recall your excitement as you mount the crest of a roller coaster, your nervous system buzzing in anticipation of the impending plunge. What makes the ride thrilling is the instantaneous flip of gravity's two sensations within your body. The sensation of your body's weight is primary during the ascent. While your heart might be in your throat, the rest of your body is thrust back and down as the car's momentum seals your body to the seat. At the ultimate moment, when the bottom drops out, your sense of bodily weight thrillingly vanishes, and for a little while you seem to be flying through space.

A thrill ride is a game with gravity—a game we've loved since our first adventures on a swing set. We begged an older sister to push us again and again so we could keep feeling the moment when our bodies changed from being heavy to being light. We enjoy that same momentary loss and recovery of the sensation of weight whenever an elevator stops or starts abruptly. These sensations of weight and weightlessness are our orienting perceptions. The feeling of being heavy tells us where down is, and the feeling of being light gives us a sense of space. These perceptions help us to stand upright.

Spatial Orientation

What keeps the body down on the planet is easier to understand than what keeps it upright. We feel rooted because gravity's downward pull gives us the experience of bodily weight. To overcome gravity and move, we must be able to perceive our spatial environment. Ida Rolf used to talk about a "skyhook." Indeed, the sky, when thought of as a metaphor for the spatial environment, is a major contributor to our upright stance. What gets us off the ground and keeps us up is our relationship to what is outside ourselves.

You can test this notion with an experiment. While standing at ease, lift one foot from the ground to a comfortable height. Then close your eyes. Concentrate on controlling your balance. Notice the degree to which you wobble, and the muscular effort it takes to keep regaining your balance. Rest a moment, and then balance again on the same leg, closing your eyes. This time focus your attention not on your body but on sounds in the distance—bird song, traffic noise. If you are doing this in an enclosed space, listen to imagined, far-off sounds, like ocean waves or church bells across town.

Compare the results of the two attempts. Most likely you were more stable and coordinated the second time. When you extended your hearing, your spatial perception counterbalanced gravity's downward pull. Your extended hearing also keyed your balance to your subcortical centers. This let you eliminate excess muscular effort. You experienced a similar phenomenon in chapter 8 when you practiced expanding your visual focus.

When you lack sufficient spatial orientation, you become so grounded that a simple action like standing on one leg takes twice the necessary effort. This is true in everything you do. You know how it feels to be so caught up with the weight of a personal or work situation that you are unable to move toward something that might lighten the load. You remain glued to your project, determined to "finish by five." Giving yourself some space by walking around the block can lift your spirits and make the work go more smoothly.

Our sense of space allows us to have goals and destinations outside ourselves. Our weight makes our bodies rebound from the earth so that movement can continue. Thus, weight and space are the inextricable yin and yang of human movement.

Your Dynamic Axis

Your posture is your ever-evolving relationship between the earth and your environment. Your body's central axis is not an abstract concept. It is a dynamic perceptual and emotional experience of the world. In describing your mood—high as a kite or down in the dumps—you are also describing your relationship to the gravitational field.

Let's review how a single posture zone influences your relationship to gravity. When tension around your pelvic floor restricts your hips, your legs and spine cannot freely adapt to gravity's demands. With your pelvis immobilized, you cannot fully ground your feet, freely extend your spine, or lift your head and heart. This limits your ability to orient yourself, so you must achieve stability in some other way, such as by gripping with your toes, belly, breath, or jaw. The resulting tension compresses your joints and restricts fascial articulations, reducing your capacity to move with ease.

Having worked through the preceding chapters, you probably have become aware of several habits that close your body in the course of daily living. Closure in any posture zone can draw your body up away from the earth or fix it too firmly down. Either way, the tension limits your orienting perceptions. If habitual closure pulls your body up and draws it down simultaneously, this curls you inward around your center.

The hallmark of healthy posture is dual orientation—the capacity to orient yourself equally well to the ground and to your surroundings. When your posture zones are free of chronic tension, you can both rest into gravity's embrace and rise up from it.

Orienting Preferences

You may have noticed that certain explorations in this book felt almost too simple to bother with, whereas others were impossibly hard. Perhaps when reaching out from an open chest or grounding through your big toe, you thought to yourself, "no big deal." Different people, however, will find different practices challenging. This is because some people relate themselves most easily to the ground whereas other people get their bearings from their spatial environment. The two orienting preferences lead to two distinct walking styles.

Earth-orienting people move with an innate sense of their bodies' weight. Their walking gait has a strong downbeat. When you watch them, you see the physical confidence that a secure relationship with gravity provides.

For people who orient themselves spatially, the concept of being grounded is foreign. These people step lightly over the ground, one step following the next in a continuous patter. Because their tensions prevent them from fully yielding to gravity, space-orienting people have little sense of their bodies' weight. This can even be true for someone who is overweight. In fact, having a poor ability to feel grounded can be an underlying reason for carrying excess weight.

Both ways of orienting have benefits. A strong relationship to the earth gives you a secure sense of personal presence and the capacity to stand firm in confrontations. Orientation to the spatial environment lets you relate to the world outside yourself or move quickly out of harm's way.

It is not yet understood how orienting preferences evolve. They may be genetically programmed or learned from our mothers' movements before we are born. They may be influenced by culture or derived from responses to traumatic events. In any case, how we orient ourselves stems from a primitive response to our environment. It is something we do with the subcortical regions of our brains. We cannot change our orienting preferences by using conscious, cortical thinking to dictate different orienting behavior. However, because strong orienting preferences can compress posture and inhibit freedom of action, it is important to find some means of modifying them. The first step is to become familiar with the sensations and movements that are associated with each orienting habit. For this we need, once again, to consider our relationship with gravity.

On the first day of geometry class you learned that a straight line is defined as the path between two points. Gravity's path through our bodies is also defined by two points. When you are standing up, your center of gravity is located approximately two finger-widths below your navel and halfway between the front and back of your body. This places it behind your intestines and just in front of the third lumbar vertebra. Martial artists have long recognized this center as the seat of physical power.

When you are sitting down, your body has a different center of gravity. This one is located just behind the upper part of your heart and in front of the spine between your shoulder blades. An infant reaches forward and up from this center on her journey from sitting to standing. The evolution of humans from standing on four legs to two can also be viewed as a journey initiated by the upper gravity center.

People who orient by means of their spatial surroundings tend to initiate

Friends

You can observe orienting preferences in action by watching reruns of the popular television show *Friends*. Phoebe, the flighty blonde, is sky-orienting. Everything about her—her speech, her lovelife, the way she thinks, even her clothing—is spatially oriented. Ross also has his head in the clouds. On the other hand, slow moving, slow-thinking Joey clearly orients himself toward the ground. He's so grounded that he's often stuck. When he knows what he wants, however, he can push to get it. Monica, too, earth-orienting, with a scrappy, down-to-earth view of things. Chandler and Rachel have more adaptable physical orientations and more versatile personalities. Both tend toward "pie-in-the-sky" thinking but readily come back down to earth.

walking from the upper gravity center. Those who orient to the ground initiate movement from the lower center. The following exploration will help you identify your preferred center of orientation by observing how you initiate your steps.

Exploration: Stop and Go

Stand where you can walk at least twenty feet in one direction. You'll be walking five or six paces forward, stopping, and then walking again. You'll repeat the start and stop several times. It's easier to sense your initiatory action if you do not have to turn around between starts.

Walk forward quickly, as if someone has called out your name. Try this several times. Be sure to stop dead after each short walk. Stop and relax as if you are going to stand there forever. Then make your next start.

Try to sense your body during the instant just before you move. Notice whether your body settles down into your pelvis and legs before you step or whether you first lift upward or forward with your chest. These subtle internal actions express your primary orienting perception. They indicate whether you derive more security from the ground under your feet or from your surroundings. Your orienting preference formats the patterns of tensions in your body. Habitual orientation to either earth or sky closes your posture to some degree.

Some of you will readily feel either the upper or lower center leading the action. Others will feel only a slight lifting of the body as they take off or a slight settling before they push forward.

If you're not sure, ask a friend to observe you. Remember, unless you stop completely and relax before each start, you may not sense your preparatory ascent or descent.

Postural shape is not the same as orientation. Some earth-orienting people have broad, open chests. Although that is part of the common space-orienting posture, you can initiate movement from the upper center even if your chest is closed. Likewise, some people with broad chests initiate movement from the lower center. You can't assess your orienting preference from your standing posture. What determines your preference is not your posture per se but the subtle activity that occurs within your body just before you move.

Both ways of initiating movement are useful, depending on the context of an activity. Many situations are best handled by walking away—by moving out into space. Other situations are best resolved by standing your ground. We all have both sets of skills, but especially under stress, we rely on our orienting preference. The goal, though, is to be adaptable. Once you have recognized your orienting habit, you can decompress your posture by cultivating sensations of the opposite orienting preference. In this way, you engage your subcortical brain to make changes that you cannot accomplish with your conscious mind.

If spatial orientation is your tendency, fostering sensations of your body's weight will help you become more grounded. Exercises that promote this include Exhaling Surrender (p. 86), Shifting Sands (p. 149), Pushing the Floor (p. 151), and Sacred Ground (p. 152).

If you tend to be earth-orienting, you can lift your posture by expanding your perception of the space surrounding your body. Exercises that encourage spatial orientation include Inhaling Beauty (p. 86), Reaching (p. 124), Sacred Touch, Living Touch (p. 131), Two-way Touching (p. 132), and Receptive Eyes (p. 164).

Nick Learns to Salsa Dance

Nick, the paramedic, is one of those people who orient themselves to the ground. During his first year of back pain, all he could do was hunker down and wait. Pain made his world shrink. Walking in the mountains was his saving grace. By drawing his perceptions up and out, the trees and peaks helped decompress his spine.

Nick has been free from pain for more than a year. It was time to try something new, but who'd ever have dreamed it would be dancing lessons? He has to admit, Carmen has him—hook, line, and sinker.

It took a few lessons for him to trust his hips and spine and to be sure the moves weren't going to set something off. Yet Carmen—who dances like a free, exotic bird—begged him to keep trying, so he hung in there. The secret was to let go. There was no controlling the salsa music, and when he stopped trying, it felt great. It was like the high he used to get from snowboarding when he was a kid.

ANATOMY OF ORIENTATION

Any muscle works most efficiently when the two ends that attach it to the skeleton are at their furthest extension before the muscle contracts. For example, your biceps muscle flexes your elbow more powerfully when your arm is extended rather than bent before you start.

This also holds true for the body as a whole. Your movement is most dynamic, efficient, and graceful when there is optimal distance between the feet and crown before you move. Correct use of your posture zones allows this lengthening to occur. Crucial to the open posture required for healthy walking is length in a specific muscle, the *psoas major.* The psoas is part of the core posture zone, but because it runs lengthwise, its main function is movement rather than stabilization.

Your psoas muscles reside deep within your abdomen. They line the front of your lumbar spine, starting from the diaphragm and passing behind your kidneys and intestines. They then cross over the front rim of the pelvis and attach to your upper inner thighs. The right and left psoas muscles are like a set of suspenders inside your body, connecting your legs to your spine.

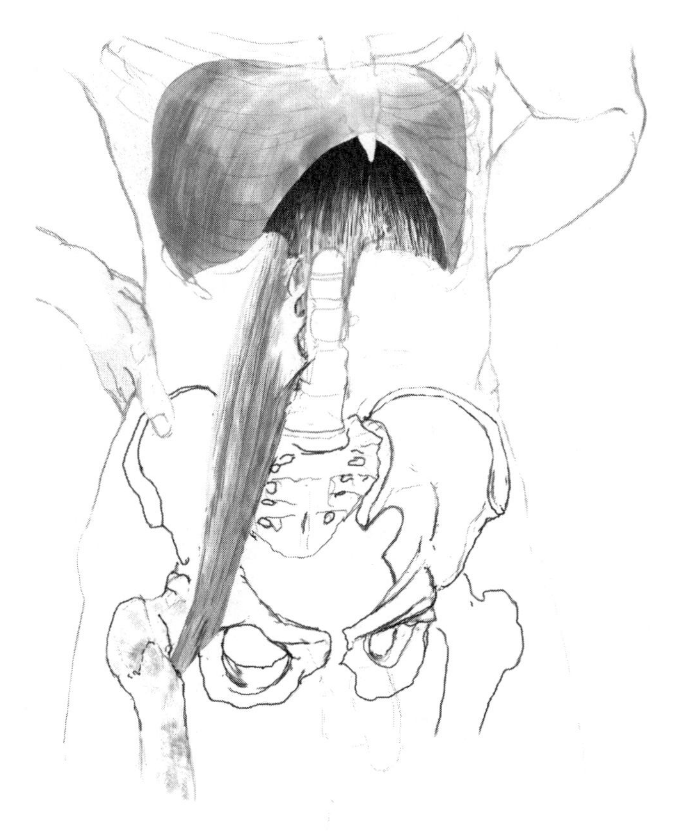

Fig. 9.1. The fascia of the crura of the diaphragm blends into the upper fibers of the psoas. This "suspender muscle" is the only muscle that directly connects your legs to your spine.

The normal action of the psoas is to bend the hip and swing the thigh forward in the course of taking a step. The right psoas and left psoas work in tandem. As one side contracts to bring the knee forward, the other side relaxes and is stretched in preparation for the next leg swing.

By raising the rib cage, healthy breathing lengthens the upper psoas attachments. Releasing tensions around the pelvic floor and hips lengthens the lower end of the psoas. When the pelvic floor, diaphragm, and inner corset function as they should, the psoas contracts to produce hip movement. However, pelvic floor tension, a short outer corset, restricted breathing, or any postural closure can make the muscle's contraction create static tension rather than dynamic action. If compression of the trunk prevents the pelvis and spine from rotating, the psoas becomes chronically short and tight. Instead of being like a set of elastic suspenders, the psoas then becomes like two rigid, stabilizing pillars. This limits the psoas' participation in walking.

Recall Sacroiliac Rocking (p. 45). When you do that exercise with attention to the slow release of your sacrum from top to bottom, you lengthen your psoas muscles. This restores their potential for dynamic activity. The following practice gives you a different way to lengthen your psoas.

Psoas Action and Orienting Preferences

A muscle can contract by drawing its two ends toward the middle or by pulling one end toward the other. If one end is pulled, the resulting action will be different than if the other end is pulled. Your *psoas* muscles in the groin can pull from either end, producing two distinctly different walking styles. Earth-orienting people fix the lower end of the psoas, so their steps draw the torso forward to meet the leg. Space-orienting people, who initiate movement from the upper gravity center, swing their legs forward to meet the trunk. It's a subtle difference, but it's obvious once you recognize it. Joey and Phoebe from the TV show *Friends* embody the two walking styles. If you're a fan of antique musicals, you will also recognize the difference as you watch Gene Kelly and Fred Astaire. In healthy walking, the psoas muscles work dynamically, without habitual fixation at either end.

Practice: Wall Traction Enhanced

You began this practice in chapter 6, where it was presented as a way to release your rib cage and shoulders (p. 126). Stand with your toes about three inches from a wall, aligning your legs so that your knees face the wall. Rest your lower breastbone and forehead on the wall. Slide your open palms up and overhead as far as you can comfortably reach. Seal the skin of your palms and fingers to the wall surface. Straighten your elbows and roll your armpits to face the wall. Rest in the stretch while you remind yourself to breathe through your lower back rib cage. Be aware of the skin on the soles of your feet. Relax, lengthen, and ground all ten toes. Seek balance through your tarsal sinus—your foot's dimple. Relax any tension around your pelvic floor.

Now, without allowing your hands to budge, slowly move the tops of your shinbones forward. This action will flex your hips, knees, and ankles. Your knees move forward two or three inches at most. Rest with this added traction for several breathing cycles.

What you should feel is a subtle elongation of your lumbar spine as your knees bend. The traction lengthens your psoas. If your arms and trunk are free of fascial restriction, you will feel as though your sacrum is suspended from your hands.

After several breaths, inch your hands higher up the wall, straightening your legs by reaching up. This gives you a new starting position. Slowly repeat the entire process, always checking to be sure that your effort is not causing closure in any posture zone.

You may find that restriction in your shoulders and upper spine prevents you from accessing the psoas. In such a case, continue practicing the stretch without the knee bends until you achieve more upper body flexibility. The traction is beneficial even if you are not yet able to achieve the full psoas stretch.

After you have repeated the traction exercise two or three times, gently slide your arms down and step back from the wall. Take a moment to let your body process the information you've just given it. When you feel settled, spend a few minutes exploring the effects of the practice on your walking. To the extent that your body can adapt to the stretch, the decompression will allow more rotary action in your spine. You may feel this as unaccustomed mobility in your spine as you walk.

As you walk, take advantage of the awareness you've gained in previous chapters. Engaging your TA will support the rotary actions of your lower spine. Engaging your serratus to support your arm swing will support the mobility of your upper spine. Accessing your peripheral vision and spatial awareness will contribute lift to your neck and take weight off your chest. Stepping into your whole heel rather than its back edge will bring your body forward over your feet and activate their spring-like potential.

Pushing and Reaching

Our two orienting perceptions correlate to two specific physical actions when we rise from sitting to standing. If you are earth-orienting, with a clear sense of your body's weight, pushing is a natural action for you. To move from sitting to standing you tend to lean your weight forward and push down into the floor with your feet.

If you orient spatially, actions that reach out feel natural. You stand up from a chair by looking out toward where you're going and reaching forward with your chest. You might even take a forward step before you're fully upright. It does not occur to you to push down on the floor to rise, nor does that action feel familiar.

If you are aware that your posture is earth-orienting, you can develop your spatial orientation by practicing actions that involve reaching out. If your body orients spatially, you can cultivate your sense of weight by developing pushing actions. Cultivating the less familiar gestures makes your coordination more adaptable and frees your joint and fascial articulations for healthy walking. The following practice encourages pushing and reaching in equal measure.

PRACTICE: FLYING TABLE ENHANCED

This practice, when carefully performed, rolls most of what you've learned into one meditation. Through it, you will practice the orienting actions of pushing and reaching, check your posture zones, and engage muscles needed for healthy walking. The choreography of this practice is the same as for the Flying Table in chapter 5 (p. 104), but the added details make it more comprehensive and powerful. Review the earlier practice before doing this one.

Position yourself on your hands and knees on a carpeted floor or mat. Have your wrists directly below your armpits and your knees directly below your hip joints. Place a folded blanket under your ankles if they are too stiff to contact the floor. Establish slow, moderate nose breathing through your lower rib cage. Release the back triangle of your pelvic floor. Gaze at the floor about twelve inches in front of your hands. At the same time, let your peripheral vision take in your surroundings.

Be aware of having equal skin contact through the fingers, palms, and heels of your hands. Draw the back edges of your armpits forward, toward the floor, to activate the serratus. Feel the contact of the floor or blanket against the skin of your shins, ankles, and tops of your feet. Balance the sensations between your hands and shins. Seek equal skin contact through all four "table legs."

Now, pushing down with your hands and feet, add a few more ounces of pressure through all four supports. If all your posture zones are open, this slight push will result in the characteristic sensation of inner corset activity.

Maintain the sensation of pushing the floor while you carefully transfer your weight to three supports. Then reach your right leg back and up. Move your leg as if the sensitive undersides of your toes are reaching out to touch something. Enliven your toes. At this point you are pushing with three limbs and reaching out with one. Modulate your efforts so that you feel you are reaching out to the same degree that you are pushing down.

Be sure to breathe steadily throughout this practice. You may find that your visual focus narrows as you attempt to stabilize your balance. Soften your suboccipitals by sustaining receptive vision and relaxing your jaw.

Smoothly transfer your weight onto two supports as you reach forward with your left hand. Imagine the skin on your finger pads seeking contact with your

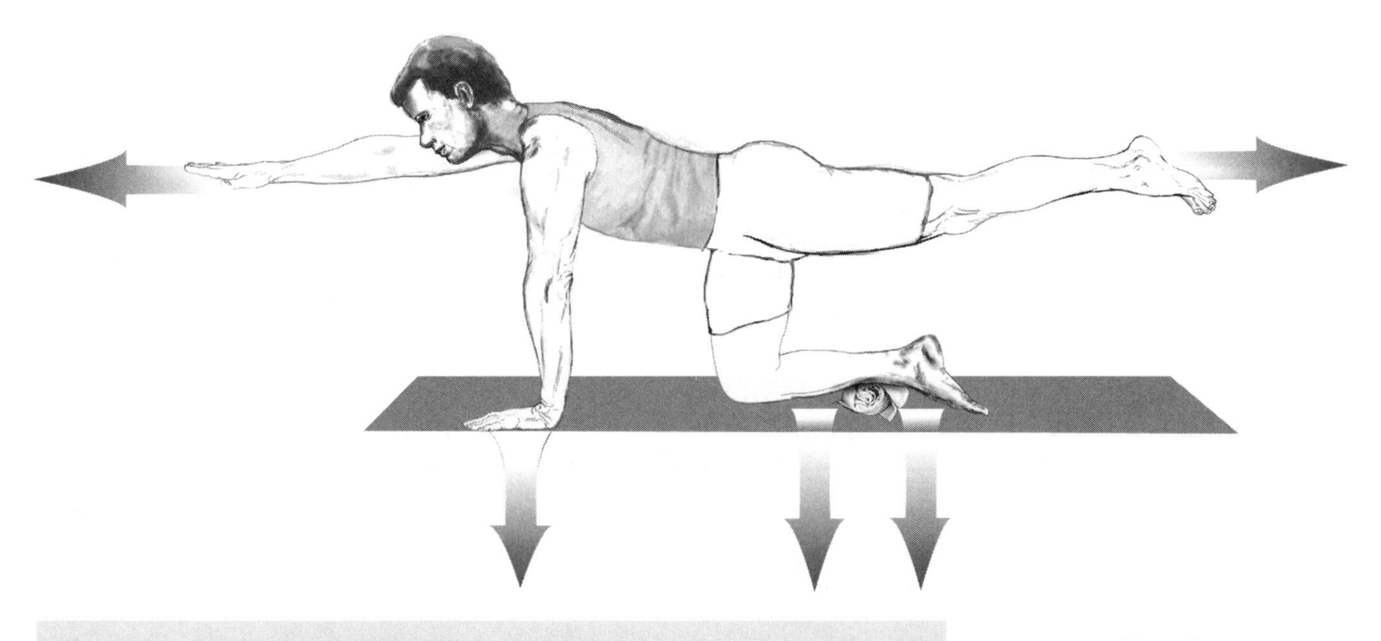

Fig. 9.2. Adding the sensations of reaching and pushing to your practice of the Flying Table helps you repattern your habitual orienting perceptions.

heart's desire. You now have two limbs reaching and two limbs pushing. Balance your efforts so that the pushing and reaching actions feel equally energetic. Let your grounded hand and shin fully feel the sensations of pushing down into the floor. Let your other hand and foot fully feel the action of reaching out. Gaze beyond your reaching hand. Sustain your actions for a breath or two and then slowly and with control return to your beginning position. Repeat using the opposite arm and leg.

Notice the difference between merely lifting your limbs as you did when you learned this practice in chapter 5 and giving meaning to your actions as you are doing this time. When you push and reach as if to touch something, you feel your muscles working in concert rather than as separate entities. Further, the opposition of reaching and pushing automatically evokes core stabilization without your thinking about it. Remember that TA contraction is a natural orienting action, one of the first things to happen when you gesture with a limb. Therefore, performing this practice as a meaningful gesture rather than as an abstract action automatically engages your inner corset. Also, by engaging your tactile skintelligence, you integrate your movement at the deepest levels of your nervous system. Practice two or three repetitions of the Flying Table each morning to help repattern your habitual orientation. Always take a moment after your practice to notice its effect on your gait.

Carmen Steps Out

"Are you sure you're well enough to go out?" Theresa worries that Carmen burns too many candles with her job and school, and now this new young man.

"I'm fine, Mama," Carmen calls from the bathroom. There's no way she'll let Nick go dancing without her. He was so uptight at first, but she could tell he liked the music. He stuck it out for three lessons while she watched his studied reserve begin to melt. Now all the other women want to be his partner.

Carmen shakes her hair to test the effect of the earrings. She's looking good. But wait a minute . . . The new blouse doesn't fit like it did in the store. She checks the size. The blouse is fine but her body looks all slouchy. What's happened? She runs through her mental checkpoints: pelvic floor released, bikini squeeze, breathing . . . but of course. She had coughed for a solid week—who knew that would take such a toll on her posture?

Carmen stretches up against the wall to restore the open feeling in her chest. It takes several minutes for the tight muscles to let go, but when she stands back, the wrinkles in her blouse are gone.

How Do Humans Walk?

Research suggests that humans have been walking on two legs for 3.5 million years, seemingly plenty of time to get it right. But you need only watch a toddler to know that walking is no simple proposition. Taking steps necessitates successive rebalancing of the segmented skeletal frame over one leg and then the other. A two-year-old sways precariously, arms outstretched, and careens forward without knowing how to stop. Stand up and try it now. Imitate your niece or nephew. The crudeness of a toddler's coordination shows his immaturity. His feet are like little sausages, his legs wobble, and his spine and arms are taut, but it's a start.

In chapter 1, you were introduced to the idea that walking should consist of movement in three planes: front-to-back, side-to-side, and rotation around the body's plumb line. To move from two leg supports to one, we, like any toddler, must shift our balance sideways. A walking style that overemphasizes this side-to-side motion is the stereotypical "jock walk."

If you watch a marching band, you can see an exaggeration of the front-to-back motion. Because their instruments must be kept steady for playing, the musicians stiffen their hips and trunk. They lean back and step with a forward-kicking motion of the knees. Soldiers march this way also, the "goose step" being an extreme example. Eyes are locked forward and necks and spines kept rigid. Legs and arms swing robotically. Such movement has a hypnotic effect that can stir school spirit or patriotism, but we'd steer clear of anyone walking this way through the local supermarket. We instinctively recognize the movement as nonhuman.

When the front-to-back motion dominates walking, the heels dig in for leverage with which to pull the body forward. This is tiring because forceful heel contact actually blocks momentum. The body must then work harder to catch up to the feet.

The rotary, or horizontal motion is demonstrated by women who walk with swiveling hips. In this walking style, the pelvis pivots around the waist, but the movement is not reflected through the upper spine. Because the rotary motion is restricted to the lower body, it catches our eye. We see it as ungainly or seductive but not truly graceful.

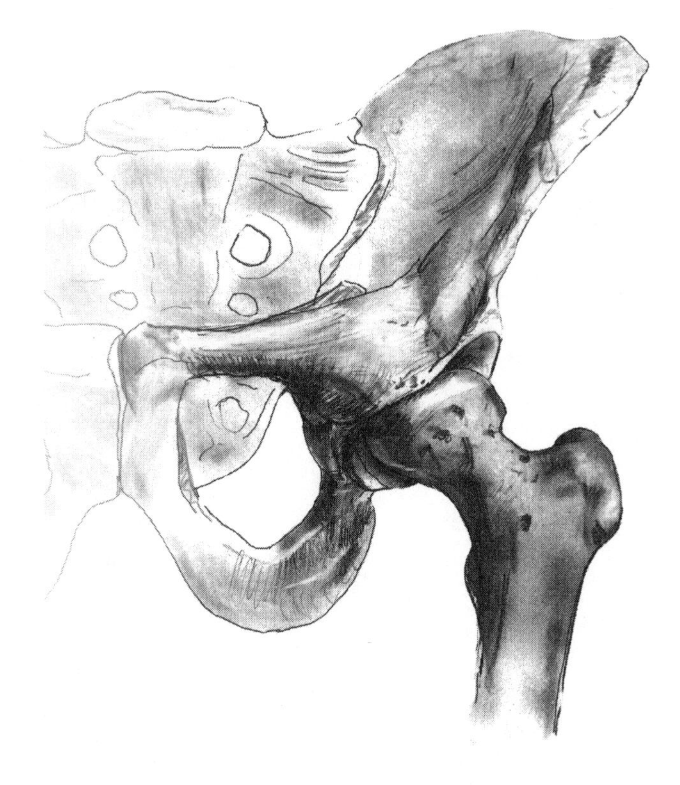

Fig. 9.3. The ball-and-socket hip joint lets your pelvis rotate as you walk.

The most natural and efficient use of our joints and soft tissues involves all three planes of motion in seamless coordination. When the three motions occur simultaneously, they interpenetrate each other like spiraling currents in a body of water. When we see human movement that has this flowing quality, our own water-based bodies respond. In our minds, we call it beautiful. Let's look briefly at the anatomical feature that allows this flowing multiplanar motion to occur.

The key to healthy walking is found in a little understood feature of the hip joint. The ball-and-socket engineering of the hip allows the thigh to move in almost every direction. The only joint in the body with greater range is the shoulder. This seems odd because conventional walking requires only that the legs swing forward and back. Rotational capacity at the hip might seem to be designed exclusively for ballet dancers or kickboxers.

The ball-and-socket design has purpose beyond moving the leg in all directions. The hip joint allows the pelvis and, with it, the whole body to move in relation to the legs. You make use of the front-to-back capacity of the joint when you bend forward from your hips. But the hip joints also let the pelvis rotate around the body's central axis. Because most people take steps by holding the pelvis still and flexing the thigh, it does not occur to us that rotation of the pelvis could contribute to forward action of the leg. In fact, the thigh and pelvis counterrotate with every step.* Pelvic motion is a natural function of the hip joint when you move from a two-legged stance onto one leg to walk. The next two explorations will help you understand this.

Exploration: Hip Rotation

Stand with your weight distributed evenly on both feet. Gradually shift your weight to the right until you are resting over your right foot. Leave your left foot touching the floor but without weight on it. Relax and let your pelvis yield onto your right hip joint. You will notice that as your pelvis settles, your right thigh rotates ever so slightly inward, to the left. The leg does this not through any muscular action but as a result of relaxation in the hip. When you are standing, internal rotation is the natural action of your thigh when your hip yields to gravity. But there's more. Notice that your pelvis has rotated very slightly to the right, toward your right leg.

Try the experiment on the other side. Gently yield your weight from a two-footed stance onto your left leg. Your left knee comes under your body by rotating toward the center while your navel turns a few degrees to your left. As a result, the belly button and knee come into line with one another.

With thigh and pelvis curving toward one another, you have shifted your central axis over the weighted leg. The counterrotation cocks the hip joint like a coiled spring, twisting its muscles and ligaments. As the joint untwists, it will lift the pelvis and contribute to forward motion in the opposite leg. You'll feel this in the next exploration.

---

*David Clark and Gael Ohlgren, "Natural Walking," *Rolf Lines* 23 (1995): 21–29.

EXPLORATION: COUNTERROTATION

Release your pelvis into your right hip as in the previous exploration. Your left foot should touch the floor passively. Rest your right hand lightly across your buttock, just behind your right hip joint. Now, without using your left leg to help, lift your pelvis back up onto two legs. In doing this, your right thigh begins to reverse its rotation, an action that impels your left hip forward. The muscles that bring this about lie deep within your right buttock. You may have felt their activity under your hand.

Repeat the experiment. This time, as your pelvis lifts off from your right hip, let your left leg respond. Let the momentum of your right hip's action drive your left foot forward into the next step.

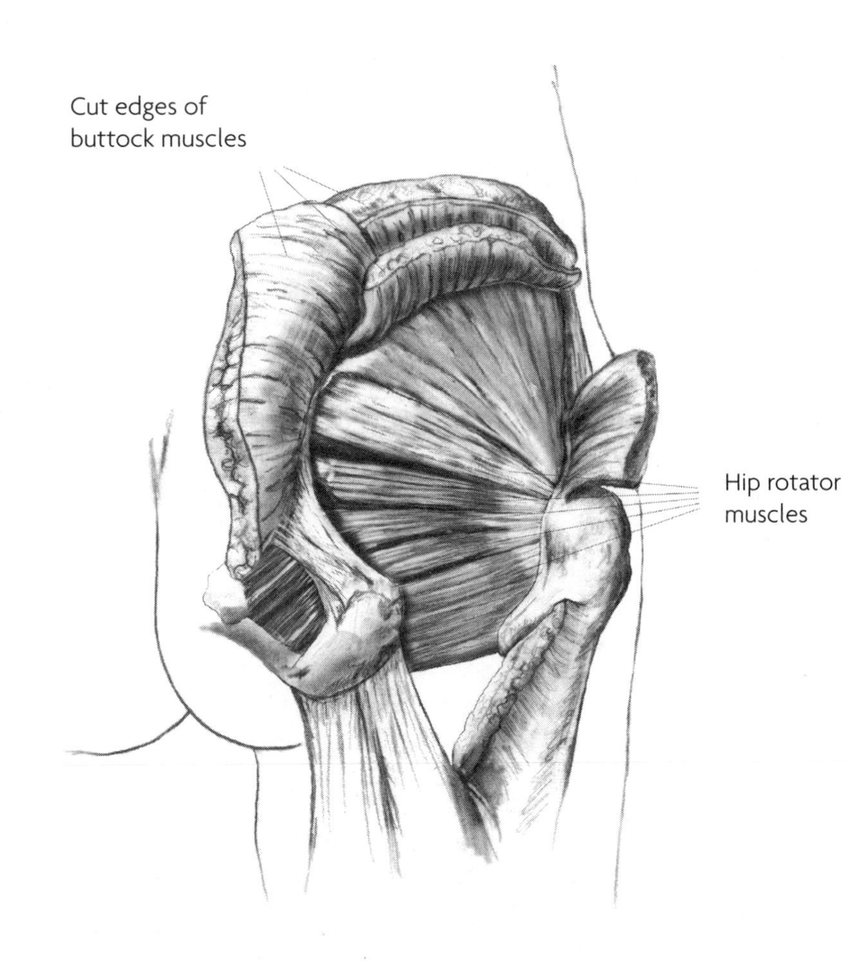

Fig. 9.4. The deep hip rotator muscles counteract gravity's inward rotation of the thigh.

Anatomy: The Mysterious Hip Rotators

The subtle winding and unwinding of the hip joint that you experienced in the Hip Rotation and Counterrotation exercises (pp. 184 and 185) is the secret of healthy walking. Along with several large muscles that operate the hip joint, there are six small ones whose primary function is to turn the thighs outward. They are located underneath the buttock muscles. This is a curious anatomical feature, because people do not ordinarily move sideways like crabs. The reason for these muscles is clear, however, when you understand that gravity's natural effect is inward rotation of the thigh. With every step, your thigh rotates slightly from outward to inward in response to gravity, then subtly outward again as the hip rotators help you resist gravity and push off from the ground.

The slight outward to inward roll of the thigh is coordinated with a slight outward to inward action (supination to pronation) of the foot as it moves from landing into push-off. Relaxation of the hip lets the weight of the body contribute to the power of the push-off. If the hips cannot relax and accept the body's weight as it shifts from leg to leg, the completion of the push-off will be interrupted by the forward-reaching action of the leg. This accounts for the common walking pattern of pulling the trunk forward with the forward-stepping leg. In healthy walking, the torso is impelled forward by the forward push of the back leg.

Because walking is so habitual, revising the way you walk can only be a gradual process. Although *The New Rules of Posture* has been leading up to this endeavor, you still need to proceed little by little, remembering that your lower brain centers must assimilate many new sensations to coordinate your walking in a way that will feel natural. The following two practices will help you cultivate healthy sensations of movement in your pelvis, hips, and spine.

Hip Opener Stretch

If your hips are too tight to feel much motion in your pelvis, you'll need to do something to open your hip joints. Structural bodywork can help, and yoga abounds in stretches for this area. The one suggested here is a simple way to start.

Lie on your back with your knees bent, legs parallel to one another, and feet on the floor. Cross your right ankle over your left knee. Clasp the back of your left thigh with your hands and draw your left knee toward your chest. You should feel the stretch through your right hip joint. Rest in the stretch for up to eight slow, moderate breaths. Make sure that you are not tensing your pelvic floor, shoulders, throat, or jaw. Repeat on each side two or three times. Then walk around to feel the increased freedom in your hips.

Practice: Pelvic Gyroscope

Use this practice to bring awareness to your hip joints and pelvis. To begin, stand comfortably with your weight evenly distributed over your feet. Relax your knees and ankles. Imagine that your crown is suspended from the sky, and that your sacrum is suspended from your crown.

Now pretend that the tip of your coccyx is a magic crayon that you can use to inscribe designs in the space around you. Begin with a simple circle. Move your crayon in a slow, smooth clockwise circle. Relax your ankles, knees, and hips. The small circular motion of your coccyx results in a generous sweep of your pelvis as a whole. Feel how your pelvis is riding on the ball-and-socket joints of your hips .

Now circle counterclockwise. Spend more time circling in the direction that feels less familiar or easy. To avoid controlling the movement with your buttocks, release the back triangle of your pelvic floor. You do not need to grip the crayon to make it move. Also relax your hands, jaw, and eyes.

Make your circle as slow, smooth, and round as feels pleasurable. The slower you go, the more you interrupt your habitual coordination. On the other hand, trying to make a perfect circle puts you in the wrong state of mind for your reptilian brain to integrate new movements. Let the movement feel good. Let it travel down into your feet and up through your spine to your smile.

After a minute or two of circling in the horizontal plane, experiment with circling front to back or up and down. Make curlicues and figure eights; you are limited only by your imagination. Feel free to put on some music because you are, in fact, dancing. Once your hips feel warm and fluid from this practice, try to sustain the sensations while you walk. For many people, just realizing that the hips are ball-and-socket joints and knowing that a certain amount of pelvic rotation is anatomically correct lets them relax the hip area enough to allow the subtle rolling motion of healthy walking.

Practice: Seated Spine Spirals

In healthy walking, the pelvis not only rotates as a whole but also twists internally. The right ilium rocks back as the right leg swings forward, and as the left leg swings back, the left ilium rocks forward. The two ilia are nodding minutely back and forth on either side of the sacrum. Luckily, you don't need to fully grasp these mechanics for healthy pelvic movement to occur. Practicing sacral rocking helps you mobilize the sacroiliac joints so that the ilia can rotate as they should. Begin by reviewing Sacroiliac Rocking from chapter 2 (p. 45).

Now, while sitting on a firm but padded chair, remind yourself of your healthy sitting and breathing cues. Arrange your feet on the floor so your thighs are parallel, and your ankles are just forward of your knees. Slowly move your right kneecap forward about an inch while allowing your left sit bone to roll back. The movement is so subtle that someone observing you would not notice it. Then slowly and smoothly reverse the movement. As your left knee reaches forward, your right sit bone rolls back. If you lightly place your fingers across your ilia, you'll be able to feel them reversing directions.

As you continue the alternating motion through your SI joints, sense the response in your lumbar vertebrae. Spend several minutes observing the subtle wave-like motion travel up through your spine. Be aware of the way that your pelvic floor diamond changes shape as the two ilia rock back and forth. Adaptability in the pelvic floor is crucial to the articulation of your sacroiliac joints, hips, and lumbar spine.

If you have difficulty feeling this motion, revise your sitting position. Your lumbar vertebrae require a neutral curve to be able to rotate as they should. The back triangle of your pelvic floor should be spacious, and your whole pelvis should be tipped slightly forward. Your lumbar spine should be gently curved, not flat. If you have a habit of tilting your pelvis back, it can help to let your pubic bone sink toward the floor. Your lumbar curve must also be well stabilized. Feel for that priceless 10 to 25 percent contraction of your inner corset.

If your spine is free enough, you'll feel your chest rotating opposite to your pelvis. But do not force your upper body to rotate. Doing this will only confuse your coordination and feel artificial. Your spine can only achieve the correct response by letting go. If these subtler movements elude you, forget about them for now.

You achieve mobility in your spine by decompressing it. You decompress your posture by orienting yourself equally to the earth and sky. Open orientation, in turn, fosters open stabilization through your posture zones.

Mika's Epiphany

"Who would have thought we'd be learning to walk all over again?" says Mika. She's trying to circle her coccyx, but her pelvis feels like a block of wood.

"Try sitting on the exercise ball," Alfredo suggests.

After Mika lets her pelvic floor settle into the ball's cushy surface, she finds it easier to circle her pelvis. She can feel sensations of movement in her hips, as if for the first time. When she stands up, she has an odd feeling of being closer to the ground. Even stranger is how it feels to walk. The looseness in her hips feels good—sexy, even. Could she walk this way in public?

An image flashes across her mind of a woman in an elaborate wedding kimono. Suddenly she's pulling boxes out of a closet. After several minutes, she holds up an old photograph.

"Alfredo, look! No wonder my hips don't move. I walk like my grandmother."

The Increments of Walking

Coordinating the actions of the sacroiliac joints, hip joints, spine, legs, and feet is too complex a task to be mastered by your conscious awareness. To cultivate healthy walking, you need to practice the elements of walking as individual sensory events. When you begin taking sequential steps, you must forget about what you've practiced and let your subcortical movement centers coordinate the sequencing.

The next three practices will offer you a repertoire of sensations, each one of which contributes to healthy walking. Practice each one separately, allowing time for your subcortical brain to integrate the movement. Do not try to coordinate the elements by analyzing how they fit together. Your analytical brain will only confuse matters and leave you frustrated.

Practice: Initiating a Step

In this practice, you will rehearse the internal orienting action that should take place an instant before you take a step. Stand with your weight evenly distributed through your feet. Take time for the skintelligence of your feet to register the ground. It's easiest to do this in bare feet, but you should also learn to sense the ground through the soles of your shoes. Be open through your pelvic floor, rib cage, shoulders, and jaw.

Gently press down into the floor with the balls of your feet while simultaneously lifting your heart. You should experience the action as a subtle elongation of your central axis, an internal gesture that moves you simultaneously down into the earth and out into the world. By decompressing your structure, the action makes room for the rotary motions of walking.

You can assist the lift of your upper gravity center by inhaling as you push down through your feet. Expand your breath equally through the front and back of your rib cage. This helps you lift your whole thorax, not just the front of your chest. Draw the back edges of your armpits forward to engage your serratus anterior muscles and broaden your upper back.

Rather than tensing your feet and toes to push down, simply deepen the contact of your soles with the floor. The downward and upward impulses should feel equal. Float up with your ribs to the same extent that you push down with your feet. Neither action should be forceful. Use only enough energy to feel a subtle two-way extension through your core.

Be aware of your favored orienting direction. If you are space-orienting, pushing down into the floor should be your emphasis. If you are earth-orienting, then lifting your rib cage is what you need to foster.

Practice: One Step

In this practice, you will take a single step by combining the hip action you felt in Hip Rotation (p. 184) with the whole body decompression you just explored in Initiating a Step. Beginning with your weight on both feet, gently yield into your right hip. Allow your right thigh to rotate slightly inward. Let your left leg be passive. Now, push down into the floor with your right foot while lifting your upper gravity center. Let this two-way action simultaneously lift your trunk from your right hip and swing your left leg forward.

In this practice, the downward push of your right foot has a slight backward vector. It can help to imagine that you're on a moving sidewalk that you operate by pushing down and back. The momentum of this action thrusts your upper center forward.

When your left foot meets the ground, your trunk is already centered directly over it. Notice also that your entire left heel contacts the ground, not just its back edge. Your right foot, the push-off foot, follows through. As you land on your left foot, the undersides of your right toes are completing their push off.

Return to the starting stance and repeat the single step on the same side four or five times. Focus on how the action feels rather than how it looks. Just as you begin to rest into your right hip, push down and back with your foot while lifting your torso upward. Land with your heart over your left foot. Let each attempt be a fresh start, without any residue from the previous try.

For the push of your foot to be successful in propelling your pelvis forward, you must release your heart area to go forward, too. If your chest is drawn down or held back, pushing with your foot will feel awkward. To move freely, your legs need the space that a lifted heart provides.

If your right heel bounces up when you push off, this indicates an imbalance between pushing and reaching. It is likely that your orienting preference is to the earth. The heel bounce is an attempt to get off the ground. Instead, focus on the lift of your chest, on extending your spatial perception, and on the backward vector of your foot as it pushes off.

Repeat the practice several times, starting with your weight on your left leg, too.

Balancing Right and Left

Many of you will find the previous practice easier to do on one side than the other. If so, you'll need to spend more time with your less coordinated side. Recall the Walking Inventory (p. 24), in which you stepped up to a ticket counter and learned that your "best foot" was actually the one that stayed behind, stabilizing your body for the step. You also may have noticed that your stronger leg gave your gait a slightly lopsided rhythm. Now, by practicing the One Step exercise, you have the opportunity to balance your two sides. This simple practice challenges all the joints involved in walking to articulate differently. It redistributes stresses through your sacroiliac joints, hips, spine, and shoulders.

You can encourage balance between your legs by reviewing Aligning Your Legs (p. 147). When you do this, imagine that you are standing on two bathroom scales. As you bend and straighten your knees, the scales should continually register equal weights. Gently correct the tendency to lean toward your stronger leg as you begin to bend your knees.

Balanced use of your legs will give your trunk better support from below, impart a smoother rhythm to your gait, and reduce wear and tear on overused joints and muscles. Balanced use of all your joints prevents you from developing chronic pain.

Practice: One Step with Rotation

This practice will add awareness of the movement of your upper body when doing the One Step exercise. To begin, check to be sure that your posture zones are open, and your spine has the elongated feeling you achieve through Wall Traction (p. 126). Then push and reach into a single step, allowing your chest to rotate a few degrees toward the landing leg. The movement occurs through letting go of your spine rather than making it move. When this feels comfortable, you can omit the previous practice.

You may be tempted to link successive One Steps into walking. If you do this, you will engage your analytical brain and impede your progress. Continue to meditate on just one step at a time. Practice with full attention for several minutes and then forget about it. Just walk with a curious attitude about the possible effects of your practice.

Practice: Forget About It

By practicing the elements of walking in small increments, you have been developing the subtle spiraling and counter spiraling impulses that should travel through your whole body as you walk. The subtle inward and outward rotation of the hip joints is at the center of this spiraling activity. However, you cannot master this flowing motion by trying to control it.

Instead, just walk. Let your subcortical brain integrate as much of the new coordination as it can. Forget about the counterrotating action of the pelvis and chest. Forget about releasing your hips. To the extent that the spiraling action can emerge, it will. Rotation of your hips and spine is your body's natural motion, but you cannot develop it by twisting your spine on purpose. You can, however, decompress your posture to give the rotations room to occur. Open your zones before you begin. Then push down and back into the floor and lift your heart.

Find specific times and places during your daily routine to tune into your walking. This can be as you take your first steps in the morning, your walk across the parking lot at work, the walk down the hall to the restroom, or your walk in the park after you've let Freckles off his leash.

Features of Healthy Walking

As you patiently practice the increments of walking as developed in this chapter, it can be helpful to notice certain features that distinguish your healthy walk from your usual habit.

First, look for your back leg to be the active one, not the front leg. The downward pressure of your push-off foot activates muscles of a fascial chain that runs from your sole up the back of your leg, through your buttock, and across your spine to your opposite shoulder. By way of this connection, the push of your foot gives impetus to a spiraling action in your trunk. This slight rotation is enough to stretch your psoas muscle, increasing its efficiency in swinging your leg forward. The dynamic push-off of your feet also tones your buttock muscles with every step, giving them a better workout than anything you can do in a gym. Healthy walking is a sure route to a shapely derriere.

Second, if your pelvis can rotate forward to settle squarely over the stepping foot, you are always in balance. Walking this way is more energy-efficient than walking with your front leg swinging out ahead. In the latter case, you spend unnecessary muscular energy pulling your body forward and must repeatedly regain your balance over your feet.

Third, by landing on your whole heel instead of its back edge, you engage your foot's built-in spring system. By widely distributing the stress of landing, you prevent strain in both feet and spine. This is how your feet are designed to function.

Finally, the coordination of pushing and reaching decompresses joints that are compressed by gravity every time you land. The gyratory motion that winds and unwinds your soft tissues absorbs the shock and releases it through the fascial system as forward momentum. The overall feel of such walking is smooth and steady, relaxed and effortless. Head, heart, and gut are always centered over the foot that bears weight. By being balanced like this, you are always "here and now." Using the hips' ball-and-socket joints correctly gives new meaning to the expression "being on the ball."

Carrying Loads

Healthy walking as described in this chapter assumes that you are walking on flat surfaces and not carrying anything in your arms. When you carry a backpack, push a stroller, drag wheeled luggage, or hold someone's hand, the motion of your upper body is necessarily curtailed. This makes your pelvis and hips move less, too. Even though rotation is restricted, you can sustain some features of healthy walking by remaining open through your posture zones.

Mika and Alfredo Learn to Walk

Mika has been showing Alfredo how her grandmother had to walk to keep from tripping over the long kimono. With her knees held tightly together, she skims over the living room floor. "My culture taught me how to walk," she says, "and yet I've never owned a kimono."

She stops, stretches her hips a bit, and then moves toward the kitchen. "This new way of moving feels like every step gives my buttocks a massage. It feels powerful . . . and a little scary. But there's something restful about it too."

"I know what you mean," Alfredo says. "It's like there's a moment of rest between steps." He walks down the hall, experimenting. "You know the pause in your breathing? It's like that, a tiny vacation."

"There's something else," he says after a while. "It makes my body feel fuller, not so narrow."

Mika looks at him. "Do you think the way you walk could be because of your . . . you know, your. . . ."

"Being gay?" he says, nodding. "I remember the day I decided to stop moving my hips. I even remember where I was. I was thirteen, and I was tired of being bullied by the boys in the neighborhood. Machismo was strong where I grew up in Chile. So after that I watched how my uncles and cousins walked. I learned to swagger . . . like a man."

The two are quiet for a while.

"It sure feels better when you stop disguising your body," Alfredo says.

Restoring Orientation

Alfredo and Mika both need better orientation to the ground. They need to develop the sense of their body's weight and to practice the feeling of pushing actions. Mika's cultural patterning keeps her from resting into the earth. In Alfredo's case, it is the trauma of his childhood and the stress of being an outcast. As they develop new, unfamiliar orientations, both will find resources for approaching their lives in more resilient ways.

Nick, on the other hand, is grounded to a fault and tends to lose his spatial orientation when he is under stress. He survived the months of rehabilitation after his surgeries and being stuck in a job he hated by staying tightly focused on pushing through obstacles. What kept him going was his love of the outdoors. The wide-open spaces kept him sane during those trying times. Now, though, life is good. A pretty girl thinks he is fine company. This is good stress, but stress all the same, and stress usually draws Nick's body inward and down. In the next chapter, he'll figure out how to handle his current stress in a different way.

10 ARTICULATE LIVING

> *We are not stuff that abides, but patterns that perpetuate themselves.*
>
> NORBERT WIENER, MATHEMATICIAN AND FOUNDER OF CYBERNETICS

Along with Alison, Nick, and Carmen, you've been experiencing your posture as the embodiment of your conflicting needs to be stable and to move. In part 1 of this book, you became aware of how your postural habits are generated and learned about the connective tissue system that connects everything within your body. In part 2, you investigated the regions of your body responsible for stabilizing your core. You discovered that stability could close and compress your posture or open and emancipate it. Part 3 showed you that the way you use your senses affects both how you stand and how you perceive the world around you.

Part 4, the current and final section, explores your body's movement. In chapter 9, you began to translate healthy posture into healthy walking. In the present chapter, you'll first expand your movement vocabulary and then review the essential practices of healthy posture. You'll examine the relationship between good posture and exercise, and you'll also see how the new rules of posture can inform your choice of a fitness program and improve your workouts. Finally, you'll review some of the body-mind connections that can turn your quest for healthy posture into a process of self-discovery.

Nick Hears His Tension

Despite his startling success on the dance floor, Nick has found healthy walking to be more of a challenge than he'd originally thought. After nearly a decade of guarding against one pain or another, it's tricky to just let go and allow the natural rotation of his spine to occur. When he's tired or irritable, his pelvis seems to tuck under of its own accord.

One night, when he'd stayed late in the lab at school, he heard his footsteps echoing in the empty hall. He could actually hear his tension—hear it before feeling it in his body. So now he listens. His old tucked-under, sideways, rocking gait produces a thud with every step, a muffled hammering. But when his spine and pelvis are rotating, the sounds have a softer, ongoing rhythm. That's when walking feels so easy, like he's a perpetual motion machine.

Becoming aware of his walking has made it impossible not to notice what other people are doing. Nick sees resilient spines in little kids and flowing motion in a few athletic types, but many people look like the only joints in play are their knees and elbows. Those folks look the way he used to feel.

Right now, waiting for his girl in the casino of their Las Vegas hotel, he doesn't see much human motion at all, but rather a chaos of blinking lights that accentuates the disembodied stillness of the gamblers huddled around the tables. It was Carmen's idea to see some shows and play a little poker. They've been dating for six months, and this is their first weekend getaway. He hopes it's going to be a good one.

Articulation

The flowing coordination of human movement depends on the joints and muscles being unrestrained by shortened fascia. A habitually closed posture makes fascial sheaths adhere to one another and this reduces articulation of the joints and soft tissue. It makes movement look and feel awkward, like poorly rendered animation.

To achieve a healthier posture, you need to release any habits that close your body. But to do that you also need to restore fluid motion to parts of your body that do not freely articulate. You do this by moving in ways that are out of the ordinary for you. Nick did it when he started learning to salsa dance, a process that took the former mountain biker out of his comfort zone and helped him relax his hips.

When you move your body through a variety of activities you use different joints. By adding variety to your movements, you make your neuromuscular coordination more adaptable. Such movements also send bioelectric impulses through your connective tissues, helping restore the adaptive gliding of your fascial planes. Variety of movement makes your body more plastic.

Research suggests that performing unusual movements contributes to intelligence and creativity* and may even lie at the foundation of the consciousness that distinguishes us from other creatures. When researchers compared the movements of various primates, they saw that chimpanzees swung through the trees with far more complex, nonstereotypical movements than did smaller monkeys. The heavier primates, our ancestral cousins, had to have enough body awareness to avoid falling by moving strategically. Smaller primates could get by with repeating the same actions over and over.†

Whether swinging through trees or sitting all day in a twenty-first-century office, repeating the same actions over and over limits your movement vocabulary. Perhaps you've noticed it limiting your perceptual horizons as well.

The following practice will help you enjoy playful, nonpurposeful use of your body. The improvisational structure of the exercise disengages your habitual ways of moving and helps restore articulation to your tissues.

Practice: Body Parts Art

Clear a space in your room so you can move six to eight feet in any direction without bumping into things. You're going to have your eyes closed, so move any furniture that could bruise your shins. Wear comfortable clothing and have your feet bare so you can clearly sense the floor. (Slippery socks on a wooden floor will keep you from feeling grounded.) To deepen your experience, wear a blindfold. This will intensify your sensations more than merely closing your eyes.

In the Pelvic Gyroscope practice (p. 186), you were invited to enhance the motion of your hips by drawing with an imaginary crayon affixed to your coccyx. For Body Parts Art, you can place the crayon anywhere on your body: elbow, nose, belly button, heel, sit bone, heart, or shoulder blade. Imagine a sphere extending to about six feet around you in all directions. All the space within the sphere is your "sketch pad." Begin moving your crayon with long, sweeping strokes. Later you can add zigzags, dots, and squiggles. You can draw from any position: standing, kneeling, squatting, or even lying down. You can move about within your sphere or stay in one spot.

Keep your crayon on whatever body part you initially select for at least three minutes. This may seem like a long time to stay involved with what your elbow

*Carla Hannaford, *Smart Moves* (Alexander, N.C.: Great Ocean Publishers, 1995), 96–107.

†Daniel J. Povinelli and J. G. Cant, "Arboreal Clambering and the Evolution of Self-Conception," *The Quarterly Review of Biology* 70 (1995): 393–421.

can do, where it can go, and how it can feel. However bored or frustrated you may become, if you continue to explore, you will break through to an unfamiliar movement or sensation. Let the rest of your body follow and respond to the wild creativity of your crayon. Vary the pace and rhythm of your movement, sometimes going very slowly. When you slow your movement, you interrupt habitual patterns and make way for new expression.

Remember to breathe. Divide your attention between your breath and the path and rhythm of your crayon. Avoid making judgments about how your movements may look. If you try to be attractive while you do this exercise, you will stifle your exploratory process. If you have a background in dance or gymnastics, avoiding self-criticism can be the most challenging part of the practice. Allow yourself to take in the pleasure of moving your body in unusual ways.

If you locate your crayon along the central line of your body, the practice becomes a sensuous dance. Explore making circles, spirals, and figure eights from your belly button, from a point between your breasts, or from the notch between your collarbones. You can even locate the crayon inside your body—at your perineum, or within your heart. Wherever you place it, let the movement be pleasurable.

If you decide to use music for inspiration, avoid playing favorite tunes and rhythms that invite you to move in too familiar ways. You are trying to evoke motions you've never done before, so play music that is unfamiliar as well. World music or ethnic fusion styles work well.

Use Body Parts Art as a morning meditation to prime your body for healthy posture during the day. In the evening, it can help you relax before sleeping. No matter how many times you repeat the exercise, you will always be able to find new movement. Once you get the feeling for it, you can work with two or three crayons at once and coordinate intricately layered movement designs.

In time, it should occur to you to add your awareness of the healthy posture zones to what you are doing. As you move in unusual ways, practice sustaining the openness of your pelvic floor, the security of your inner corset, the constancy of your breath, and the skintelligence of your hands and feet.

Movement and Feeling

Whether or not we are aware of it, our movement is always accompanied by sensation, because moving and sensing are linked within our nervous system. This means that restoring articulation restores sensation to your body as well. The return of sensation to a suppressed area can be upsetting.

Pleasurable sensations can be as difficult to integrate as painful ones. If your only awareness of physical pleasure has been in association with intoxicating substances or sex, the simple pleasure of physicality may take some getting used to. This is all the more true because Western culture has curbed the public expression of physical pleasure for so many centuries.

Media images of rich and famous people can influence our view of physical beauty. When our physiques do not match up with current bodily fashion, we may deny the pleasure of our own bodies. Shunned body parts include big feet, wide hips, small breasts, and large noses, any of which might be fashionable in another time and place. Women's bodies are especially vulnerable to fashion, although men, too, can be made to feel inadequate about their bodies.

Restored sensation can be stressful, too, because sensing may remove an illusion of invisibility. If you have ever felt shame or fear about any part of your body, you probably managed your feelings by withdrawing your awareness from that part. In effect, you made that part of your body disappear by immobilizing it.

Sometimes, rediscovery of movement sensations in the chest, throat, or pelvis can cause someone to revisit unpleasant memories of sexual innuendo or abuse. Should this occur to you, you may need a period of work with a counselor to feel safe releasing the tension that may have been your only protection during trauma. Our bodies often retain their defensive tensions long after they are needed, and it is not unusual for the release of those tensions to release cleansing tears as well. Holistic approaches to healing trauma are listed in the appendix.

Orienting Yourself by the New Rules

The basic premise of *The New Rules of Posture* is that poor posture is neither something you are born with nor a life sentence. Posture, good or bad, is the result of the collection of habits that have evolved along with your life experiences. This is the second new rule of posture: your posture is the product of the ongoing perceptual activities through which you orient yourself to your world.

When your body is dually oriented to the ground and your spatial field—when you are making equal sense of earth and sky—the muscles of posture impart optimal length to your body. This lengthening prepares the muscles of movement to contract dynamically. The harmonious coordination of stability and movement gives your actions power and grace.

The preparatory lengthening should recur, over and over, between successive actions. When you orient yourself more to one direction than the other, you diminish the security that orienting in both directions provides. Dual orientation is the arbiter of graceful and efficient movement. It is healthy posture in action.

Your orientation and your posture zones are interdependent. Adaptability in the zones facilitates dual orientation. Dual orientation prevents the zones from overstabilizing. Recall that the zones are regions of muscle and fascia that are roughly perpendicular to your vertical stance. They are like valves or doors that control your vertical alignment. Because fascia runs uninterrupted through them all, closure in one affects the others.

When any zone is unnecessarily engaged in stabilizing your body, you diminish your perception of the ground, your surroundings, or both. When your feet are tense or your pelvic floor is closed, you do not fully experience the ground. With no feeling of being supported by the earth, you cannot accurately perceive the weight of your body. If you do not sense your weight pushing into the earth through your feet when you walk, your legs and spine lose both power and grace.

Clenching your teeth or tongue, focusing tightly with your eyes, or gripping with your hands all reduce your awareness of the space around your body. Diminished spatial perception, by limiting your sense that it is possible to reach out, inhibits your freedom to move into the world. Your awareness of chronic or recurring tension in any posture zone should signal you to exchange that tension for open stability. You achieve this through having tone in your inner corset and through renewing your perceptions of ground and space.

Such self-awareness is the essence of the first new rule of posture. You gradually, patiently replace any stabilizing tensions that close your body with your newly created sense memories of open stability and open orientation.

Healthy Posture Practices

When you realize that your posture is a perceptual phenomenon, it becomes clear that you can't improve it without addressing your perceptions. The practices in this book have been designed to help you do that. For that reason, they are of little use if performed by rote. Their effectiveness depends on you fully feeling the sensations that are being evoked.

The following review can serve as a program for daily renewal of your posture.

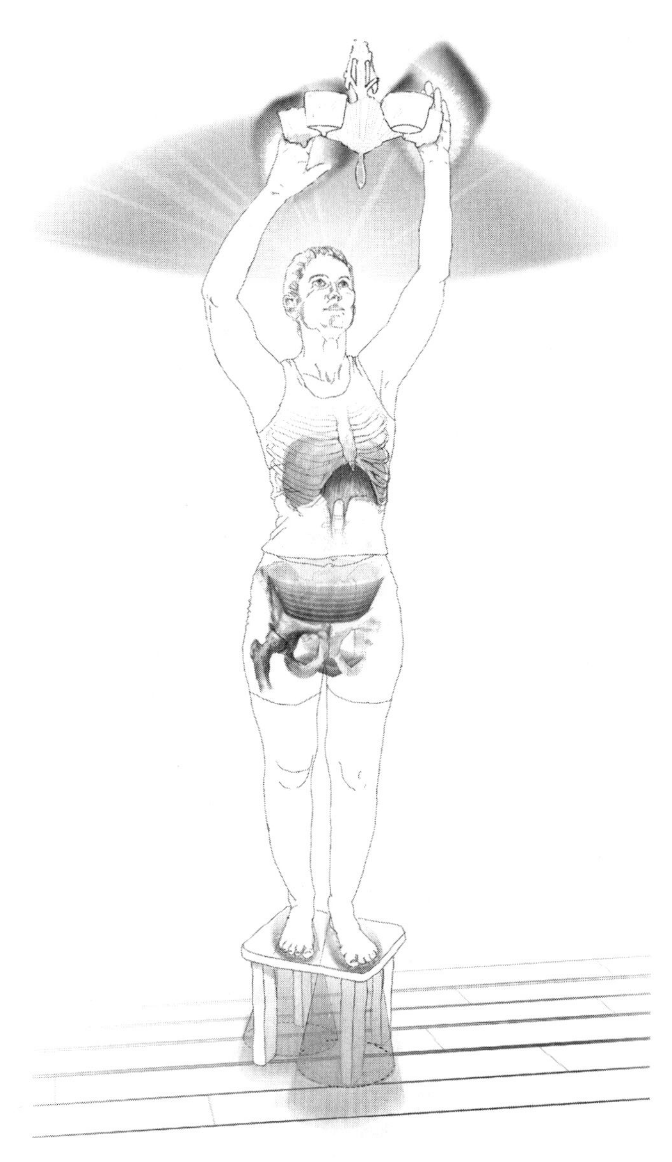

Fig. 10.1. Alison found it easy to polish the chandelier after she understood how all six posture zones contributed to the way she used her body.

- Body Parts Art (p. 197). This dance-like improvisation deepens your physical consciousness and helps you mobilize parts of your body that you don't ordinarily move.
- Sacroiliac Rocking (p. 45) mobilizes your sacroiliac joints to allow full articulation of your pelvis and lumbar spine in walking.
- Curling and Arching (p. 50) evokes motion between your individual vertebrae.
- Breathing in Gravity (p. 87) reminds you of the features of healthy breathing and healthy sitting. Integrate breathing awareness into all of the other practices.
- Flying Table and Flying Table Enhanced (pp. 104 and 180) combine awareness of breathing, the pelvic floor, and the inner corset; the pushing and reaching gestures of orientation; and strengthening the muscles involved in walking.
- Wall Traction and Wall Traction Enhanced (pp. 126 and 178) stretches your shoulders and rib cage, elongates your psoas muscle, and decompresses your spine.
- Footprints on the Wall (p. 142) enhances articulation in the joints of the feet.
- Aligning Your Legs (p. 147) helps you align the joints of your feet, ankles, knees, and hips. Once understood, this practice can be integrated into Wall Traction.

- Shoulder Blade Pulses (p. 118) and Handprints on the Wall (p. 120) align the shoulders and rib cage and activate the serratus anterior muscle. When they are understood, both can be integrated into Flying Table.
- The facial explorations in chapter 8 (starting on p. 158) help you release tensions in your jaw, eyes, and neck, making possible the dynamic balance of your head. Incorporate the awareness gained through these explorations into all other practices.
- One Step and One Step with Rotation (pp. 190 and 192) fosters the development of healthy walking.
- Walk while meditating on the healthy posture cues that have been most meaningful to you. Your greatest resource for sustaining healthy posture is healthy walking. Each of your ten thousand to twenty thousand steps each day can either sabotage or reinforce your new posture habits.

Walking the Zones

As increasingly urbanized Westerners, most of our walking is confined to shopping malls, hallways, and parking lots. Our gaits are constrained by walls, objects, or people. Such barriers conspire to reduce arm swing and limit push-off, reducing the power with which we stride into the world. Yet sometime during each day there are moments when each of us can walk without being encumbered by bags, briefcases, phones, or to-do lists. Turn those moments into healthy posture practice sessions by focusing on one zone at a time throughout the day.

As you walk, avoid thinking about the precise coordination of your arms, legs, and spine. Healthy walking develops not by thinking about what you're doing but by savoring the perceptions that foster fluid movement. Cycle your awareness through the posture zones. Feel how landing on your whole heel cushions the impact of your steps. Be aware of spaciousness through your pelvic floor. Feel the nanosecond of rest as your weight releases into your hip joint. Feel how mild activation of your inner corset contains your core, supports the rotation of your lumbar spine, and lets you breathe in a way that lifts your rib cage.

To emphasize your spatial orientation, let your peripheral vision perceive the shapes and colors of your environment as you move through it. Notice how a release of tension in your eyes releases tension in your neck and allows your head to float.

Experience the weight of your body being received by the earth with every step. Imagine the ground coming up to welcome your feet. Sense your legs pushing the ground behind you as if you were on a moving sidewalk. Feel how this action activates your buttock muscles.

The more you practice feeling the sensations of healthy walking, the smoother and more effortless walking becomes—like riding a wave and being the wave at the same time.

EXPLORATION: ACCELERATION

Being in a hurry exaggerates your orienting preference. If you tend to be earth-orienting, you hunker down, plowing through the thick of things like a fullback through the other team's line. If you are the space-orienting type, you are more likely to skim over the ground as if ready to take flight. In either case, your posture suffers. This exploration will help you prevent the rush of daily events from sabotaging your posture.

Establish your current version of healthy walking. Then, very gradually, increase your speed up to the point where you begin to lose dual orientation. The moment you sense your body closing, slow down and begin again. In time, you can coach yourself to move rapidly without the closure that so often accompanies being in a rush.

Alison's Marathon

Alison's first marathon attempt had ended abruptly after eighteen miles. She was an experienced runner and she'd trained hard and well, yet there she'd been, doubled over, panting in the street.

This year, though, things would be different—she could feel it. She'd found a book about a regimen that included meditation, diet, and a training method that her macho running partners made fun of. They called it "nose running." It involved training only as hard as she could while maintaining steady breathing through her nose. In the beginning, embarrassingly, her runs slowed down almost to a walking pace. But she'd read that nasal breathing would increase her respiratory efficiency, and now, after five months, her persistence is paying off. Who would have believed that her breathing rate would drop as her runs got tougher? No more gasping and hyperventilating. Instead she ran easily, with plenty of energy to devote to sustaining *her posture. She felt her feet pushing back against the road and enjoyed the scenery as it grazed her peripheral vision. Her body seemed to operate of its own accord, without effort. She must have attained that performance zone that elite athletes talk about. Just now, at the fifteen-mile mark, she'd left her training partners in the dust.**

Fitness

Healthy posture is not a substitute for exercise. In fact, lack of flexibility can prevent you from experiencing the sensations of healthy posture, and lack of strength and stamina can keep you from sustaining it. Although there can be no doubt that exercise contributes to health, exercise, in and of itself, doesn't guarantee healthy posture. The type of workouts you choose to do and how you do them can make all the difference to your posture. When you exercise you should do the following:

- Choose activities that accentuate the perceptual orientation you need to develop.
- Include both strength-building and stretching exercises.
- Vary repetitive, linear movements with activities that include rotation.
- Exert yourself only to the extent that you can sustain open posture.
- Stay aware of your body while you're working out.
- Choose activities that give you pleasure.

We will look at each of these below.

Adaptable Orientation

If you tend to find your orientation from the ground, you can develop spaciousness in your body by learning dance styles such as tango or swing that move you around the dance floor in wide arcs or by playing golf or other sports that demand spatial awareness. Ballet, with its emphasis on reaching out through the limbs, also develops lift.

A space-orienting person can develop groundedness through the earthy movements of jazz or hip-hop dancing or by playing team sports like basketball that require pushing actions. The movements of tai chi employ a good balance of both orientations, as does the martial art aikido. In con-

*The book Alison read was *Body, Mind, and Sport* by John Douillard. It's listed in the bibliography.

trast, wrestling or boxing draw the body into its center, away from both earth and sky.

Strength and Flexibility

Athough strength and flexibility are not mutually exclusive, our genetic heritage tends to endow each of us with more of one than the other. People with well-muscled structures tend to have more strength, while those with lighter frames tend to be more flexible. Human nature attracts us to activities that take advantage of our assets. Flexible people enjoy stretching, while people with dense musculature avoid it. For healthy posture, however, you need a balance of strength and flexibility. If you are naturally strong, you need to engage in exercise that accentuates flexibility. If you are flexible, you need to build strength.

Nonrepetitive Motion

The diagonal arrangement of our musculature affirms that human movement should occur in gentle arcs and spirals, like the movement of water. Any regimen that trains the body in single planes of motion reduces the articulation of joints and soft tissues and undermines the natural flow of movement. For example, fitness machines do this. By failing to respect the curvilinear design of the musculature, such training can actually create fascial restriction and build muscle mass on top of poor posture.

When you perform the same movement over and over, your body consciousness diminishes. With less awareness and less tissue adaptability, it can be easy to establish a vicious circle of injury, immobility, and compensating tissue restriction. Repetitive movement is like water flooding a streambed, gradually eroding the ravine.

If you love the speed and athleticism of running or cycling, however, you don't have to give them up. You do need to counteract their risks with activities that involve engaging your body in a wider variety of movements. Try volleyball, basketball, or martial arts. Take up dancing, swimming, rock climbing, or yoga. Adaptable coordination is as important to your fitness as strength and flexibility. The more you move your body in different contexts, the more agile you become.

Exertion

Energetic people need the exertion of a good, hard workout to counteract the stress of sitting down all day at school or work. If your idea of fun is a ten-mile run or a two-hour flow yoga class, you'll need to modify your workout at first to embody changes in your posture. Until your new habits are established, reduce the speed and intensity of your workout by 20 percent or so, enough to let you remain mindful of your orientation and posture zones.

A good guide is the steadiness and pace of your breathing. When your effort is so great that you must breathe through your mouth, you diminish your respiratory efficiency and also compress your core and close your shoulders and chest. Nasal breathing slows your respiration and heart rate and stimulates full use of your diaphragm. In time, like Alison, you'll find that nasal breathing helps you reach your peak performance.

Modulating your exertion during exercise helps you develop the habit of noticing what effort does to your body during daily living. Excess effort of any kind, mental or physical, usually provokes closure of one zone or another. Pursing your lips, gripping your palms, pushing your belly out, or closing any other zone indicates that you are not feeling stable. Use that moment as an opportunity to exchange closure for open stability. By following the first new rule of posture in this way many times, for many months, you can form new habits for responding to challenging situations.

Body Awareness

Although rare individuals seem to have been born with beautiful posture, most of us have to work at it. Exercise alone is not sufficient. In fact, many people who exercise daily have poor posture. The woman who has such beautiful form in the yoga studio walks to her car with heavy heels and rounded shoulders. This is where your understanding of healthy posture gives you an advantage. By working out with awareness, you increase the likelihood that you'll incorporate the effects of your exercise into your daily life.

For a workout to benefit your posture, you must stay present in your body while you exercise. Many people seek to save time by reading while they work out on an exercise bike or by watching television while they walk on a treadmill. When you constrict your visual field to do this, you tense your eyes, suboccipital muscles, shoulders, and entire spine, compressing your posture. Although exercising in this manner improves heart rate, burns calories, and builds muscle tone, it also strengthens existing postural habits, thus diminishing both your adaptability and your consciousness and increasing your risk of injury. You cannot achieve healthy posture with your mind and body on autopilot.

Your posture derives from how you move. So changing how you use your body as you go about your daily routine will change your posture. You need simply to notice that how you move makes a difference and decide that it is a difference worth cultivating.

PLEASURE

It's simply true that if you choose exercise you enjoy doing, you're more likely to keep at it when life gets hectic. Enjoying your workouts has another benefit. As you'll recall from the Simple Pleasure exploration (p. 23), pleasure automatically makes your body feel more open and fluid. Pleasurable sensations activate the refined coordination of the reptilian and mammalian parts of your brain.

Movement Disciplines

Movement disciplines devoted to body-mind integration include Dance Meditation, Body-Mind Centering, and Continuum Movement. Each enhances body awareness, encourages the body's natural curvilinear motion, and encourages the pleasure of embodiment. All three are listed in the appendix.

CLASSES AND TEACHERS

A caveat for taking part in any exercise class is to be aware of the way that being present in a group can influence your self-awareness. Your teacher's urging, combined with a natural inclination to keep up with others in the group, can cause you to over-stabilize. Narrowed visual focus, held breath, or a tensed pelvic floor are common responses to class situations, each leading you to strengthen a poor habit. Group workouts can also have a hypnotic quality that may diminish your self-awareness. To counteract this effect, practice some of the exercises at home, taking time to remember your healthy posture cues. Then, when you go to your class, your internal coach will keep your body open during the workout.

Ask your instructor about the extent of her training. Certification as a fitness instructor should involve a minimum of five hundred hours of training. Notice how the teacher interacts with her students. A responsible teacher will ask class members about any injuries or weaknesses before the class begins.

Pilates and Yoga

The early twenty-first-century fitness scene is dominated by the growing popularity of two exercise disciplines, one ancient and one developed relatively recently. Both yoga and Pilates acknowledge the uniqueness of individual body imbalances and seek to correct them through body awareness and alignment. Both address strength as well as flexibility.

Yoga is a group of spiritual practices that originated in India around the beginning of the first century AD. The aspect of yoga best known in the West is hatha yoga, a series of exercises or poses practiced mainly for mental and physical health.

Yoga teachers who have been trained in the style of yoga developed by B. K. S. Iyengar are particularly well equipped to teach in a manner that fosters healthy posture. The Iyengar system focuses on details of joint alignment and muscular balance. Built into the Iyengar method is an understanding of how dual orientation activates core strength to stabilize the body in an open way. Because of its emphasis on alignment, this method is a good foundation for more active yoga styles. Although flowing yoga styles build stamina and aerobic capacity, they can overwhelm the precise body awareness necessary for changing habitual posture. On the other hand, when healthy posture is established, the stress of a fast-paced workout can be an effective way to challenge your new habits.

The Pilates method was developed in the early twentieth century by Joseph Pilates as a way of rehabilitating wartime injuries. The work involves free exercise done on floor mats and the use of spring-weighted equipment. In time, the method became popular with dancers and athletes. Pilates emphasizes the development of the core musculature as the center of the body's power. Instructors who have embraced recent research on core stabilization teach the importance of maintaining a neutral lumbar curve during workouts. When taught in this manner, the Pilates method effectively strengthens inner core musculature. Some Pilates instructors, however, may train the lumbar spine to flatten. This tends to activate only the outer core muscles and can reinforce a closed postural pattern.

Neither Pilates nor yoga engage your body in combined planes of movement. To encourage your body's natural spiraling motion, you should vary either program with an activity that involves curvilinear motion. Try belly dancing or tai chi.

Your body is not just designed to move, it needs to move. Proper movement is as critical to your health as good light, clean air, and nourishing food. People commonly tell themselves that unless they have at least half an hour to work out, it's not worth doing. In fact, five minutes of activity, if performed with attention and mindfulness, is certainly better than none. Five minutes of the yoga Sun Salute, five minutes of tai chi, a five-minute walk—those few minutes can be enough to interrupt old habits and strengthen new awareness. Five minutes of activity can remind your senses how good it feels to be present in your body. Also, when it becomes an established routine, a five-minute workout can grow into ten, displacing that second cup of coffee. After that, who knows what you might do?

Sin City

From the moment they hit Las Vegas Boulevard, Carmen was lost in the barrage of glamour. She was entranced by every entertainment ad, wanted to eat at every restaurant, play the slots at every casino, and gape at every shop window.

By Sunday morning, after twenty-four hours on the town, both of them are tired. Nick wants a change of pace, a hike to see some petroglyphs outside of town. "It'll be a cool contrast to all this glitter," he tells her.

But Carmen wants to pick out gifts for friends at home, and she has her heart set on a brunch show with gospel music. "Look," she says, pointing to a flyer, "it's a family, and they've been singing together their whole lives." Her voice has a whining tone that she doesn't like but can't seem to stop.

Nick feels himself withdrawing. He stands at the entrance to a familiar cave and watches his heart grow still in a way that isn't kind. Carmen stares out the window at the phony Eiffel Tower and tries to steady her breathing.

"I'll be back in five," he says, forcing himself not to slam the door.

He walks out to the parking lot. Sun glints off some palm trees. The hot desert air presses against his skin, but the natural sunlight is oddly soothing. The wide sky opens his body, relaxing him so that he can see the situation in a different light. In trying to show Carmen a good time, he'd gotten caught up in the hubbub and lost touch with both her and himself. Maybe she'll never be a hiking buddy. Maybe "buddy" is entirely the wrong concept.

It's simple triangulation, he realizes. Navigating their relationship is like finding his way in the mountains. If he can find three points of reference, he can know where he is. By reaffirming his sense of ground and space, he can find his center, find Carmen, and with her help, keep the space between them free of static.

Back inside, he finds Carmen doing her yoga stretches.

"Hey," he tells her. "It's stupid to try doing everything in one weekend. C'mon, we can still make that gospel show. We'll have that desert adventure some other time."

By now, you've probably become aware of the underlying theme of this book: it is as much about heightening body consciousness as it is about improving posture. Body consciousness helps you remember that life is experienced through your body. An open and adaptive body furthers an open and adaptive approach to life. Healthy posture doesn't just look and feel better, it also opens your attitudes toward and responses to situations and people. Perhaps then, the new rules of posture can be simplified into a single piece of advice: Be present in your body as you interact with your world.

Your Walk is Your Story

Just as you recognize other people by the way they walk and others recognize you in the same way, your walk also can help you with your self-study. Walking is your body's signature. Just as your handwriting can be more or less legible, your walk can be more or less graceful, depending on your mood and circumstances. How you stabilize and orient yourself throughout a day changes your rhythms, your displays of energy, and your use of space.

By tuning into the quality of your walking during daily life, you experience your body both practically, in terms of physical usage, and philosophically, as the expression of your being. The following suggestions will help you augment your awareness of the connection between your various walking patterns and your states of mind.

Exploration: Your Best Walk

Notice the physical features of your walk when you're doing things that make you happy. Notice your orientation and what's happening in your posture zones; feel the flow of your movement. Then describe how your best walking corresponds to your emotional state: are you centered, grounded, open, contained, energetic, assertive, or peaceful?

Notice how your clothing affects the way you walk. If you're a man, compare your posture in a suit and tie with how you stand in casual slacks or baggy

Saturday jeans. If you're a woman, compare the effect of a miniskirt with that of a long flowing one, heels with flats, tight jeans with easy fitting ones. Notice the effects of your make-up, hair, and jewelry. Notice which apparel evokes your healthiest posture. Then practice feeling those sensations no matter what you're wearing.

Exploration: Your Worst Walk

Notice how you walk first thing in the morning on a day when you'd rather have slept in. Perhaps, with your eyes still gazing inward, your feet shuffle across the floor, moving you into the day with as little body awareness as possible. Not wanting to be fully present can make you resist feeling the ground or avoid being aware of the space around you. This can happen at any time of day.

Observe your walk when you're distracted, exhausted, feeling angry or resentful, holding yourself together, or doing something you'd rather not be doing. Assume one of these moods and then walk around your living space. Describe the mood in terms of what happens to your grounding and spatial perception and what happens in the core of your body. Notice how your frame of mind affects the energy, timing, and sound of your steps. By identifying the physical features of your mental state, you gain a measure of choice over both your physical expression and your mood.

Exploration: Walking Your Way out of a Funk

When you're unable to think positively or are just bone tired, it is common to reverse the polarities of healthy posture. In such situations, you can use your frame of mind as a signal to amend your postural orientation or release closure around your central line. While continuing about your business, select one zone to be aware of and put just 10 percent of your awareness there. You might choose breathing into your lower ribs, engaging your inner corset, expanding your vision, or awakening the skintelligence of your hands. Along with a change in your body, you'll likely sense a slight lifting of your funk or glimpse an option you couldn't see before.

When you notice a positive shift in your mood, you are feeling the emotional resonance of your postural change. When you do this, you key in to the subcortical mammalian brain that mediates your emotional responses to the world. By registering the difference in emotional coloring, you help recode your physical behavior within this primitive brain region. By making this body-mind connection again and again, you build sustainable postural transformation.

WALKING IN THE REAL WORLD

Recall the Stabilizing Actions exploration in chapter 1 (p. 30), when your walk was affected by an intimidating person. Associating with such a person on a daily basis, as in a work situation, can make you lose your ground, compress your space, and limit your articulation. Instead, let the person's presence remind you to restore your sense of ground or space, to breathe steadily, and to engage your stabilizing inner corset. By cultivating healthy posture, you can transform both your view of the person and his or her view of you.

Transforming your posture may involve making some adjustments in your established relationships as well. When we are connected with others, we may unconsciously blend our rhythms and movements with theirs. If your partner walks with a heavy heel strike, as so many people do, it can be tricky to cultivate new patterns of your own when you're walking together. Experiment with letting your rhythm be in harmonious counterpoint with your partner's, rather than in unison.

The heart of posture is our relationships with others. How we think other people view us influences how we stabilize our bodies, breathe, stand, and regard others in return. This aspect of improving your posture can be challenging to confront. It would be unreasonable to expect yourself to be able to assume more open physical attitudes in all your relationships right away. Start by practicing with neutral relationships—the kind you have with the checker at the grocery store. A simple exchange at a checkout counter is an opportunity to interact with someone from your new open orientation.

Gospel Brunch

Nick had figured that the Vegas club scene would be all wrong for gospel music, but to his surprise, he's spent most of the morning praising the Lord with a hundred other tourists. Evidently, there's no taking the spirit out of the gospel sound.

Near the show's end, the MC invites a dozen newlyweds onto the stage to celebrate. Carmen is on her feet in an instant. "C'mon," she whispers to Nick, "Who's going to know?" Yet he hangs back. It's one thing to take a few dancing lessons, another to put yourself on display.

Now Carmen is dancing near the lead singer, in front of some people who look too shy to do anything more than bob up and down. Carmen lets the music swim through her body, lets it turn her cells into rhythm and praise. Nick feels proud as he watches her and not a little envious of the easy way she occupies her body. With thunderous applause, the audience demands one more song. "What the heck," he mutters, and bounds up the steps onto the stage.

Healing Your Posture

Taking good care of our bodies can be a daunting task and learning about them an overwhelming one. There seems no end to what there is to know about our bodies because anatomists, biophysicists, medical researchers, somatic psychologists, and movement specialists are constantly discovering new information. There can be so much to know, sense, and attend to that we may long for blissful body ignorance.

An ancient Sufi teaching can put our frustrations into perspective. The story describes reality as being comprised of eighteen thousand universes. We humans inhabit a tiny speck in just one of the universes, and what we know about our speck could fill a spoon. Yet, compared to the complexity of all that, the teaching says, the human body is vastly more complex. This suggests what scientists are discovering daily: it is as likely that we have untapped potential within our bodies as it is that we use only a small percentage of our mental capacities. To use ourselves well by honoring the body's design can only bring us closer to unlocking our physical potential.

Maintaining healthy posture requires a lifelong commitment to your relationship with gravity. A powerful partner when we learn how to interact with it, gravity is a formidable adversary when we fail to acknowledge its influence. Because it took decades to develop our habitual ways of orienting ourselves, it only makes sense that evolving new ways of being in our bodies should require a few years of sincere attention. As we coach ourselves toward healthy posture, we'll need to summon the qualities of any good teacher: patience, intention, focus, the ability to offer gentle encouragement, and knowing when to let go and begin again. Using these attributes to develop a healthy relationship with gravity helps us practice them in relation to life in general.

Healing your posture is a process of self-discovery—mental, emotional, and physical. Your patient and consistent cultivation of healthy body usage prepares you for the deeper healing that can take place when you're under mental or emotional stress. When you're moving to a new home, meeting a deadline, or working through a relationship, your recognition of postural closure or loss of orientation gives you an opportunity to respond to challenges in new ways. When you pass through such crises with efficiency and grace, you know transformation is happening.

AFTERWORD

EXPLORE THE NEW RULES OF POSTURE, TOGETHER

A powerful way to experience the program outlined in this book is to share it with a friend. Better yet, work through the book with a small group of people. You will boost your awareness enormously by meeting regularly to practice the exercises and share your experiences. We make our best progress in any endeavor with the support, encouragement, and protection of others.

So many of us have been shy about posture, assuming that there is nothing we can do to change it. By working together in a group, we can gently uncover our negative feelings about our bodies. Being in a group also lets us tap into a deep source of postural habits—our beliefs about how other people view us. For such group work to be beneficial, a pledge to maintain an atmosphere of trust and safety is required. The group you create should be a place in which to explore possibilities without fearing judgment.

We live in a culture that denigrates the body by regarding it as either a sexual object or a power object. There is little indication that mainstream culture respects the body's intelligence or its capacity to transform. Those of us who have experienced our bodies' healing wisdom need to band together for encouragement and support.

Be sure to visit my website, www.newrulesofposture.com, for up-to-date information, new articles, video content, and the opportunity to join a forum of like-minded people.

APPENDIX

THERAPEUTIC RESOURCES FOR HEALTHY POSTURE

This section contains contact information for institutes of structural bodywork, movement therapy, and body-mind approaches for working to overcome the effects of trauma. These organizations train practitioners to facilitate personal transformation through physically oriented exploration. You can contact any of these organizations to find a teacher or practitioner in your area.

Aston Patterning
www.astonenterprises.com
Gentle bodywork, movement education, and ergonomic considerations combine to help clients find integration of body, mind, spirit, and environment.

Body-Mind Centering
www.bodymindcentering.com
Transformative experience through movement education and hands-on repatterning. Experiential study of anatomical, psychophysical, and developmental principles leads to understanding how the mind is expressed through the body and the body through the mind.

Bodynamic Analysis
www.bodynamicusa.com
This body-oriented psychotherapy focuses on removing mental and physical blocks to healthy human connections by working with the interactions between tone in specific muscles and their corresponding psychological functions.

Continuum
www.continuummovement.com
Private and group sessions provide a context in which students develop sensitivity to the subtle movements of life, from breath and the fluid movement of tissue to patterns of interactions with other people.

Dance Meditation
www.dancemeditation.org
An integrated movement meditation system for self-regulation and self-healing. The process enhances body-mind integration through explorations of self with self, self with others, and self with the Divine.

Guild for Structural Integration
www.rolfguild.org
Structural bodywork following Ida P. Rolf's original ten-session protocol to release the body's structure from lifelong patterns of tension.

Hakomi Therapy
www.hakomiinstitute.com
Body-centered, somatic psychotherapy addressing the hidden core beliefs that shape relationships, self-image, and life directions.

Hellerwork Structural Integration
www.hellerwork.com
Enhanced body consciousness through structural bodywork, movement education, and dialogue on emotional themes.

International Association for Structural Integrators
www.theiasi.org
A professional association whose membership is open to practitioners trained at any of fourteen schools that espouse the teachings and philosophy of Ida Rolf. The website has a list of certified SI practitioners.

ISMETA
www.ismeta.org
The International Somatic Movement Education and Therapy Association maintains a professional registry of practitioners of various somatic movement disciplines.

Rolfing Structural Integration
www.rolf.org
Structural alignment through bodywork and movement education following principles inherent in Ida P. Rolf's original teachings.

Other Resources for Healthy Posture

Chapter 3

The Balans Chair
www.sitbalans.com
This "kneeling chair" seats the pelvis at the correct angle but puts pressure on the knees. Although this chair fosters a neutral lumbar curve, it leaves the feet ungrounded and can be awkward to get in and out of.

Bucky Natural Comfort
www.bucky2.com
This buckwheat cushion called Baxter is ideal for adjusting your sitting position in car seats and elsewhere.

The Swopper Chair
www.swopper.com
The design of this chair, which was developed in Germany by an osteopath and an engineer, promotes an open angle at the hip and an appropriate lumbar curve. Its unique spring system allows the body to move while seated.

The ZackBack Chair
www.yogaback.com
Developed by a physical therapist, this chair with an adjustable back support promotes diaphragmatic breathing, stabilizes the sacrum, and allows the lumbar spine to lengthen.

Chapter 4

The Buteyko Method
www.buteyko-usa.com
This method of breathing education works to control the symptoms of asthma by normalizing breathing.

Somatic Experiencing
www.traumahealing.com
A naturalistic approach to the healing of trauma, SE works with the neurological mechanisms that are overridden when survival behavior does not adequately discharge the high levels of energy aroused during traumatic events.

CHAPTER 7

Posture Control Insoles
www.posturedyn.com
These slim shoe inserts are designed to evoke a muscular response that corrects posture. Feet and body are strengthened by the improved mechanics of the feet rather than weakened by restricted motion, as can be the case with conventional orthotic devices and arch supports.

Nike Free Running and Walking Shoes
www.nike.com
The foot bed design and flexible soles of this line of Nike shoes elicit the foot's natural mechanics and foster healthy use of foot and leg muscles.

CHAPTER 8

CranioSacral Therapy
www.craniosacraltherapy.org
This gentle hands-on method for enhancing the functioning of the central nervous system is effective for a wide range of medical problems associated with pain and dysfunction.

Holistic Dentists
www.holisticdental.org
This is an association for dental care as it relates to the health of the whole person.

BIBLIOGRAPHY

Agneessens, Carol. *The Fabric of Wholeness*. Aptos, Calif.: Quantum Institute Press, 2001.

Anderson, Ron. *Stretching*. Bolinas, Calif.: Shelter Publications, Inc., 2000.

Bertherat, Therese. *The Body Has Its Reasons*. Rochester, Vt.: Healing Arts Press, 1989.

Bond, Mary. *Balancing Your Body*. Rochester, Vt.: Healing Arts Press, 1993.

Bradley, Dinah. *Self-Help for Hyperventilation Syndrome*. Alameda, Calif.: Hunter House, 2001.

Brill, Peggy. *The Core Program*. New York: Bantam Books, 2001.

Brourman, Sherry. *Walk Yourself Well*. New York: Hyperion, 1998.

Calais-Germaine, Blandine. *Anatomy of Movement*. Seattle: Eastland Press, 1993.

Chaitow, Leon, et al. *Multidisciplinary Approaches to Breathing Pattern Disorders*. Edinburgh: Churchill Livingstone, 2002.

Cohen, Bonnie Bainbridge. *Sensing, Feeling, and Action*. Northampton, Mass.: Contact Editions, 1993.

Cranz, Galen. *The Chair*. New York: W. W. Norton & Company, 1998.

Dart, Raymond. "Voluntary Musculature in the Human Body: The Double Spiral Arrangement." *The British Journal of Physical Medicine* 13 (1950): 265–68.

Deutch, Ronald M. *The Key to Feminine Response in Marriage*. New York: Random House, 1968.

Donkin, Scott. *Sitting on the Job*. Boston: Houghton Mifflin Company, 1986.

Douillard, John. *Body, Mind, and Sport*. New York: Three Rivers Press, 1994.

Egoscue, Pete. *Pain Free*. New York: Bantam Books, 1998.

Farhi, Donna. *The Breathing Book*. New York: Henry Holt and Company, 1996.

Feitis, Rosemary. *Ida Rolf Talks*. Boulder, Colo.: Rolf Institute, 1978.

Ferrington, D., and Mark Rowe. "Cutaneous Mechanoreceptors and the Central Processing of Their Signals: Implications for Proprioceptive Coding." In *Proprioception, Posture and Emotion,* edited by David Garlick, 56–69. Kensington, N.S.W., Australia: University of New South Wales, 1982.

Frank, Kevin. "Tonic Function: A Gravity Response Model for Rolfing Structural and Movement Integration." *Rolf Lines* 23 (1995): 12–20.

Fried, Robert. *Breathe Well, Be Well.* New York: John Wiley & Sons, Inc., 1999.

Fried, Scott M. *The Carpal Tunnel Helpbook.* Cambridge, Mass.: Perseus Publishing, 2001.

Godard, Hubert. "Intrinsic Movements: Interview with Aline Newton." *Rolf Lines* 20 (1992): 42–49.

———. "Reading the Body in Dance, a Model." *Rolf Lines* 22:3 (1994): 36–41.

Godard, Hubert, et al. "Motion ed E-Motion in Oncologia." In *Psiconcologia,* edited by D. Amadori, M. L. Bellani, P. Bruzzi, P. G. Casali, L. Grassi, G. Morasso, W. Orru, 875–81. Milan, Italy: Masson, 2001.

Goldfarb, Lawrence W. "Why Robots Fall Down." *The Feldenkrais Journal* 9 (1994): 5–14.

Gracovetsky, Serge. *The Spinal Engine.* New York: Springer-Verlag, 1988.

Grossinger, Richard. *Embryogenesis.* Berkeley, Calif.: North Atlantic Books, 1986.

Hannaford, Carla. *Smart Moves.* Alexander, N.C.: Great Ocean Publishers, 1995.

Iyengar, B. K. S. *Light on Pranayama.* New York: The Crossroad Publishing Company, 1985.

Juhan, Dean. *Job's Body.* New York: Station Hill Press, 1987.

Langevin, Helen M., and Jasan A. Yandow. "Relationship of Acupuncture Points and Meridians to Connective Tissue Planes." *The New Anatomist* 269 (2002): 257–65.

Lee, Jennette. *This Magic Body.* New York: Viking Press, 1946.

Levine, Peter. *Waking The Tiger.* Berkeley, Calif.: North Atlantic Books, 1997.

Maitland, Jeffrey. *Spacious Body.* Berkeley, Calif.: North Atlantic Books, 1995.

McHose, Caryn, and Kevin Frank. *How Life Moves.* Berkeley, Calif.: North Atlantic Books, 2006.

Myers, Thomas. *Anatomy Trains.* Edinburgh, Churchill Livingstone, 2001.

Newton, Aline. "Basic Concepts in the Theory of Hubert Godard." *Rolf Lines* 23 (1995): 32–43.

———. "Breathing in the Gravity Field." *Rolf Lines* 25 (1997): 27–33.

———. "New Conceptions of Breathing Anatomy and Biomechanics." *Rolf Lines* 26 (1998): 29–37.

———. "Posture and Gravity." *Rolf Lines* 26 (1998): 35–38.

Ohlgren, Gael, and David Clark. "Natural Walking." *Rolf Lines* 23 (1995): 21–29.

Olsen, Andrea, and Caryn McHose. *BodyStories*. New York: Station Hill Openings, 1991.

Povinelli, Daniel J., and J. G. Cant. "Arboreal Clambering and the Evolution of Self-Conception." *The Quarterly Review of Biology* 70 (1995): 393–421.

Richardson, Carolyn, et al. *Therapeutic Exercise for Spinal Segmental Stabilization in Low Back Pain*. Edinburgh: Churchill Livingstone, 1999.

Rolf, Ida P. *Rolfing*. Rochester, Vt.: Healing Arts Press, 1989.

Rothbart, Brian A. "Medial Column Foot Systems: An Innovative Tool for Improving Posture." *Journal of Bodywork and Movement Therapies* 6 (2002): 37–46.

Schleip, Robert. "Fascial Plasticity—A New Neurobiological Explanation." *Journal of Bodywork and Movement Therapies* 7 (2003): 104–116.

Schultz, R. Louis, and Rosemary Feitis. *The Endless Web*. Berkeley, Calif.: North Atlantic Books, 1996.

Speads, Corola. *Ways to Better Breathing*. Rochester, Vt.: Healing Arts Press, 1978.

Swayzee, Nancy. *Breathworks for Your Back*. New York: Avon Books, 1998.

Upledger, John, and J. Vredevoogd. *Craniosacral Therapy*. Chicago: Eastland Press, 1983.

White, Arthur. *The Posture Prescription*. New York: Three Rivers Press, 2003.

Wilson, Frank. *The Hand*. New York: Vintage Books, 1998.

Wise, David, and Rodney Anderson. *A Headache in the Pelvis*. Occidental, Calif.: National Center for Pelvic Pain Research, 2003.

Zacharkow, Dennis. *Zackback Sitting*. Rochester, Minn.: Zackback International, 1998.

INDEX

arm swing, 28, 90, 125, 179, 202

back pain, 55, 62, 67, 80, 92, 94, 95–96, 101, 108, 110, 125, 135, 139
balance, 25, 141, 149–50, 152, 156, 163, 172, 191
  60/40 balance, 64–65
  central axis, 26, 27, 73, 144, 155, 173, 184
  postural sway, 37–38
brain
  cerebral cortex, 130
  limbic system, 130
  reptilian brain, 130, 153
  subcortical centers, 130, 163, 172, 174, 176, 189, 212
breathing
  air hunger, 81, 83
  asthma, 79
  Buteyko Method, 79, 218
  carbon dioxide, 79–82
  chronic hyperventilation syndrome, 80–82
  crura of diaphragm, 76, 77, 159, 177
  diaphragm, 18–21, 39, 42, 55, 63, 75–77, 78, 83, 85, 109, 159, 177
  mouth breathing, 78, 159
  nose breathing, 78–79
  overbreathing, 80–82
  paradoxical breathing, 80
  respiratory pause, 85–86
  scalene muscles, 20, 77, 127
  shallow breathing, 21, 73, 78
  ujjahi breathing, 89

carpal tunnel syndrome, 42, 128
core, 27, 93, 103, 118, 177
  bearing down, 76, 109
  core stabilization, 95, 105, 107–10, 159, 181, 208
  external abdominal oblique, 95
  inner corset, 93–94, 96–97, 102–4, 106–7, 159, 181
  multifidi muscles, 94
  outer corset, 94, 95
  psoas major muscle, 177
  transversus abdominus (TA) muscle, 77, 89, 93–97, 103, 181
CranioSacral Therapy, 161, 219

dowager's hump, 41

emotions, 21, 25, 27, 28, 32, 49, 73, 74, 90, 103, 110, 114, 125, 130, 150, 211–12 ergonomics and sitting, 67–69

face, tensions in
  eyes, 127, 156, 157, 159, 162–65, 167, 200, 202, 206
  jaw, 156, 160, 161, 167
  nose, 157, 159
  suboccipital muscles, 157–58
  temporal mandibular joint, 156
  tongue, 158–59, 167, 200
fascia, 38–44, 48, 56, 75, 84, 93, 98, 108, 120, 127, 136, 157, 158, 193, 197
feet
  abductor hallucis muscle, 145, 146
  bunions, 140, 144, 145
  flat feet, 140
  flexor hallucis longus muscle, 145
  orthotics, 146–47
  pronation, 139
  stance foot, 137–38
  supination, 139
  tarsal sinus, 138
  walking foot, 137–38
Fuller, Buckminster, 36

gravity, 5–6, 8–9, 36–37, 60, 69, 171–72, 186, 213

hands, 114–15, 116, 117, 120, 127, 129
  touch, 114, 115, 129, 130–32
headache, 56, 79, 161
hip joints, 58, 65, 183–84
  hip rotator muscles, 185–86
  hip tension 27, 186

hyperventilation. *See* chronic hyperventilation syndrome *under* breathing

Iyengar, B. K. S., 208

Kegel, Dr. Arnold, 58, 99
knees, 137, 140, 145, 147–48, 151

laptop computers, 128
lifting, 76, 108, 133

muscular armor, 22

neck
  atlanto-occipital joint, 157
  tension in, 20, 30, 42, 56, 67, 123, 125, 156, 161–62

orientation, 6, 150, 155, 167–68
  ground orientation, 150, 152, 173, 174, 176, 204
  spatial orientation, 167, 172, 176, 179, 202
orienting centers, 173–75

pelvic diamond, 58, 64–65, 188
  anal (back) triangle, 58, 64, 98, 148
  perineum, 58
  urogenital (front) triangle, 58, 98
pelvic health, 63
pelvis
  anococcygeal ligament, 59
  anterior superior iliac spine, 46, 57
  backward pelvic tilt, 61, 92
  forward pelvic tilt, 61–62

ilia, 44, 46, 57
ischial tuberosities, 58
ischium, 57
pelvic floor, 58, 97, 109, 188
pubic bone, 46, 57
Pilates, Joseph, 208
planes of movement, 29, 182–83, 208
posture zones, 8–9, 40, 42, 73, 155, 168, 188, 200, 201

reflexology, 136
repetive motion injuries, 127
Rolf, Ida, ix, 41, 136, 147, 172

shoulders, 115
clavicle, 116
scapula, 116
serratus anterior muscle, 119–23
tension in, 28, 126
thoracic outlet, 127
trapezius muscle, 117–19
winged scapulas, 122
skintelligence, 129, 131, 132, 151, 181, 189
spine, 29, 60
coccyx, 44, 58, 59, 98
kyphosis, 60
lordosis, 60
neutral lumbar curve, 61, 62
sacroiliac joints, 44–48, 57, 62, 187
sacrum, 44–45, 46, 49, 56, 57, 69
scoliosis, 139
spinal discs, 55, 60, 62, 77, 95
stability, 6–7, 93, 109, 123, 155, 167, 195, 200
Structural Integration, 41

tensegrity, 36

urinary incontinence, 59, 93, 110

yoga, 79, 89, 186, 208

BOOKS OF RELATED INTEREST

BALANCING YOUR BODY
A Self-Help Approach to Rolfing Movement
by Mary Bond

ROLFING IN MOTION CD
A Guide to Balancing Your Body
by Mary Bond

ROLFING
Reestablishing the Natural Alignment and Structural Integration of the Human Body for Vitality and Well-Being
by Ida P. Rolf, Ph.D.

THE ALEXANDER TECHNIQUE
How to Use Your Body without Stress
by Wilfred Barlow, M.D.

THE BODY OF LIFE
Creating New Pathways for Sensory Awareness and Fluid Movement
by Thomas Hanna

THE BODY HAS ITS REASONS
Self-Awareness Through Conscious Movement
by Therese Bertherat and Carol Bernstein

APPLIED KINESIOLOGY
Muscle Response in Diagnosis, Therapy, and Preventive Medicine
by Tom and Carole Valentine with Douglas P. Hetrick, D.C.

WAYS TO BETTER BREATHING
by Carola Speads

Inner Traditions • Bear & Company
P.O. Box 388
Rochester, VT 05767
1-800-246-8648
www.InnerTraditions.com

Or contact your local bookseller